About the Autl

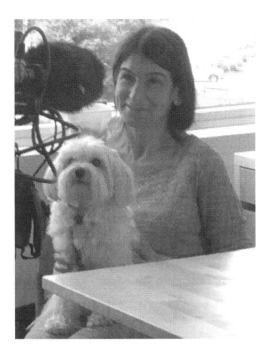

Nancy Zucker, PhD, is a clinician, researcher, and teacher at Duke University School of Medicine, where she founded and directs the Duke Center for Eating Disorders. Dr. Zucker is an Associate Professor in the Department of Psychiatry and Behavioral Sciences. She is the author of numerous professional publications and is an author of the upcoming revised practice guidelines for the treatment of eating disorders from the American Psychiatric Association. Dr. Zucker's major clinical and research interest is in understanding how to help young people develop a healthy awareness of their bodies' signals and learn how to match these to actions that allow them to flourish. Her research and clinical work has been featured on ABC's "Nightline," the Wall Street Journal, the New York Times, Time, and other major news outlets.

Table of Contents

To all the moms and dads in my parent groups whose crucial, creative, and wise insights have helped this program to evolve over the years; and, a heartfelt thanks to my mom and dad – for too many reasons to name.

Acknowledgements

I wish to thank Lisa Story, Ph.D., for her perceptive and insightful editorial comments. Her contributions were vital. It has been an honor and a pleasure working with her on this project. I also wish to acknowledge Laura Weisberg, Ph.D. whose perceptive insights throughout the years have helped me to evolve in my thinking in more ways than she realizes.

Welcome.

NOTE: We wrote this introduction section to give you some background information about the manual you are about to read. If you are anxious to get right to the skills, go ahead and start reading STEP ONE and come back here when you feel less pressed. If not, read on....

Greetings. You have just picked up a skills manual designed to give parents tools to manage your child's illness when your child is struggling with an eating disorder. This book will also be helpful for parents who are concerned your child or loved one may be developing eating disorder symptoms (or weight and shape concerns). How? Well, this book focuses on giving you three sets of tools. First, we teach you how to manage your child's disorder. Next, we teach you helpful coping strategies (strategies that we feel are missing in your child and made him/her more likely to develop an eating disorder). Finally, we help you and your child practice these coping strategies together. Our goal is not only to improve your child's symptoms, but also to make you and your family more confident and skillful in handling life's challenges so there is less likelihood of troubles returning.

Skills Taught in this Program
•   Effective Parenting Styles
•   Behavior Management
•   Self-parenting
•   Healthy Eating
•   Emotion Regulation
•   Communication
•   Healthy vs. Unhealthy Perfectionism

We feel this broad range of skills is very important. Our goal is for you to feel confident in your role as parents. We want to help you feel confident in your home environment and help your children develop in a healthy manner. By achieving this, we not only help to get rid of the disorder in the short term, we also help ensure the disorder does not come back. Our basic approach is to view eating disorders as coping strategies. Your child's disorder helps him or her to cope in some manner. Our job is to figure out how the disorder helps him/her cope and to teach more effective coping strategies so your child no longer needs the disorder. While we do this, we help your child not perform her/his unhealthy symptoms. Finally, we role model the healthy coping strategies ourselves as this helps to convey how important we think they are (and makes it so we are not hypocrites – which is far from desirable). Before we begin, let's talk about how this program developed.

How did this skills manual develop?

This program was developed in the eating disorders program at Duke University Medical Center following years of work with families who had a child with an eating disorder. It may be helpful for you to understand my thinking in the development of this program, so make yourself comfortable, I tend to get enthusiastic (some would say "long-winded") when I talk about this, so I may go on for a bit.

Much of my initial training in the treatment of eating disorders occurred while I was working at an inpatient hospital unit that specialized in eating disorder treatment. During that time, one of my many jobs was "meal monitoring." This meant it was my job to supervise a room full of patients with eating disorders and make sure they ate all the food in their meal plan without hiding, destroying, smearing, or finding other creative ways of not eating their food. Boy, was that tiring! However, after doing this for several years, I developed some strategies that made the process a lot easier.

This experience led me to think about two things. First, I thought, if I am so exhausted doing this, how in the world can parents do this? I only have to do this one meal a day. Parents may have to do this several times a day depending on their child's age and stage of illness. Furthermore, although I care greatly about my patients, they are not my children. This task would be incrementally more challenging if this was my child! Thus, I felt I needed to develop a way to teach parents these skills that I'd learned. But I needed to do more than that. I had to increase their support while they helped their child. Finally (and perhaps most importantly), I needed to give parents their confidence back.

Eating disorders totally throw parents off balance. Parents who were thinking they had been doing a pretty good job of raising their children suddenly feel frozen, not knowing which way to turn. Thus, through this program, I had to help parents get their confidence back. After all, it's not parents that are the problem. The eating disorder is the problem. Parents are part of the solution.

I've worked with families for many years. Through this work—I can tell you from the bottom of my heart—I have come to know some of the most fantastic people I have ever met. Unfortunately, they often don't think so. They blame themselves for their child's disorder and continue to dwell on what they could have done differently. It was important for me to help parents realize that this is not true and to help them feel good about themselves again (or maybe for the first time). Thus, my goal in creating this program was to find a way to teach parents skills to manage their child's disorder, skills to help parents get their confidence back, and skills to help create a healthy home environment.

Where did the skills in this book come from?

How did I select the skills that parents needed? Well, first I drew from my personal experience of working with hundreds of families whose child was receiving treatment for an eating disorder. I thought about the skills that parents need to manage this disorder. I added to this personal experience by reading and reviewing research from several different areas. First, I reviewed the treatments for eating disorders that have been shown to be effective. I took from these treatments the elements that I felt would help parents. But I didn't stop there. I also looked at treatments that have been effective in treating other childhood disorders, such as childhood anxiety, depression, or attention deficit disorder. I also took from these approaches the parts that I felt would help parents who have a child with an eating disorder and adapted them so these approaches could meet the specific needs of parents who have a child with an eating disorder.

And then I went a bit further. I added a little sugar and spice. Basically, I figured that skills are much easier to learn and problems much easier to approach if we can laugh our way through things. Having a child with an eating disorder can be one of the most painful and upsetting things a family can experience. Unfortunately, when we are really upset, we are not very effective. I don't know about you, but I sure think more clearly when I am calm.

Blah, blah, blah. OK already. Does it work? Give us the bottom line here. It's almost time for next mealtime.

Zucker ©2016

Does it work?

Parents think so. Here are some things that they have to say:

> "I don't know what I would have done without this program. I have learned so much and feel so much stronger."
>
> > \- parents of an adolescent child with anorexia

> "Attending this program was one of the best things me and my husband have ever done. I don't think there is anything that could be more helpful for my child."
>
> > \- parents of an adult child with bulimia

In their opinion, this program was essential for the management of their child. But don't believe me, here are the results from a survey they completed.

Survey of Parent Satisfaction with Group Parent Training: Results from 16 Families

	Strongly Disagree	Mildly Disagree	Mildly Agree	Strongly Agree	Not Sure
1. The parent training group was helpful in teaching me how to manage my child's eating disorder.	0 %	0 %	0 %	100 %	0 %
2. The parent training group was essential for the improvement of my child.	0 %	0 %	9 %	91 %	0 %
3. I have used the skills learned in the group in other areas besides the eating disorder.	0 %	0 %	9 %	91 %	0 %
4. The group has helped me to become a better parent.	0 %	0 %	0 %	100 %	0 %
5. I feel more confident in my parenting skills as the result of the group.	0 %	0 %	18 %	82 %	0 %
6. I would recommend this group to other parents.	0 %	0 %	0 %	100 %	0 %
7. My child would not be doing as well if I were not in this group.	0 %	0 %	18 %	82 %	0 %
8. Being in this group has helped to decrease the stress I feel as a result of this disorder.	0 %	0 %	18 %	82 %	0 %
9. Being a member of this group has taught me to take better care of myself.	0 %	0 %	36 %	64 %	0 %
10. I take better care of myself since participating in this group.	0 %	0 %	45 %	55 %	0 %
11. I can better handle stressful situations as a result of this group.	0 %	0 %	18 %	82 %	0 %
12. Other people have noticed the changes in me as a result of participating in this group.	0 %	0 %	64 %	27 %	9 %
13. I frequently use the skills taught in the parent training group.	0 %	0 %	36 %	64 %	0 %

In addition, we are currently conducting research studies to investigate how well this program works compared to other programs. The National Institute of Health and the National Eating Disorders Association have both provided funding to further study this program. If these important health organizations are willing to invest in the program, there must be something to it!

Why is it called "Off the C.U.F.F.?"

That is actually an excellent question. (As an aside, I found over the years that parents have lots of questions. Parents, you know who you are. To address these questions, at the end of every chapter, I have a "frequently asked questions section."). Now, back to your question. Off the C.U.F.F. is the style of parenting you learn in this program. This style of parenting guides you in the implementation of all the skills you learn. There have been numerous research studies that examine the type of parenting style that is most effective in promoting the health and well-being of children. This research has taught us that a "FIRM AND SUPPORTIVE" parenting style predicts less substance use, less disordered eating, less risky sexual behavior, less depression, and makes your children CEOs of major corporations (hmm). Thus, it makes a lot of sense to make this parenting style the foundation of our program. What exactly is a firm and supportive parenting style? Well, it's an "Off the C.U.F.F." style! Don't worry, we'll get there in Part I. Just keep reading…. (For your information, C.U.F.F. stands for Clear, Undisturbed, Firm, and Funny).

> Uh, before we start, can I ask a question? Why do you call it "Off the C.U.F.F.?" No offense, but I don't see how that has anything to do with eating disorders.

A Strategy for Approaching This Book

We want to give you a road map of where you're heading. We will repeat this roadmap at the beginning of every step so you can monitor your progress along the journey. This will also help you to stay mindful of where you started and how far you have come (I find parents like to overlook these things and just focus on how far they have to go). Warning, I want you to read this while thinking to yourself, "Geez, I am certainly going to learn a lot." (This is preferable to the alternative which is what I find parents usually do: "She's got to be kidding. This is a lot of information.")

FOREWORD. You are here.

Get a nice hot beverage. Decide on a comfortable location in your house (please create a favorite corner if you don't have one already. You will need this corner throughout the program). Pick a quiet time of the day when no one is around and read this foreword to introduce yourself to the program. I have found that the #1 problem I run into with parents is that they do not stop and learn. If I had a dime for the number of times parents call in crisis, and I counsel, get them through the situation, and get them to read a section and they say "Boy, I wish I would have read the manual before that happened." But wait, I'm preaching to the choir. You ARE reading. Stop reading right now and go to your chosen support person (i.e. spouse, friend, family member – more on this in Chapter 1) and tell them how important it is THAT HE OR SHE READS AT THE SAME TIME YOU READ. This is the #2 complaint I have from parents: their support person (spouse, friend, sibling) is not in there with them. They need to be. It helps your child, it helps you, and it helps your support person. Families get really stuck when both parents aren't on the same page. By participating, it makes your chosen support feel both more confident and more important. This is **so** important that every lesson has two homework sheets: one for you and one for him or her. OK. Go find him/her. I'll be here when you get back.

TIP BOX
Do nothing yet but read.
You need to have an understanding of what you will be doing before you jump in.

Chapter ONE: Understanding Your Journey.
Repeat STEP ONE (the chair, the beverage), but this time if your spouse or support has not been reading, he or she owes you a present; an expensive one. That should do it. Read Chapter 1: Understanding Your Journey. This section gives you some information about eating disorders and how we view the treatment of eating disorders. You are introduced to the idea of eating disorders as coping strategies. As such, we will have you complete a guide that has you pinpoint the coping strategies your child needs to strengthen, the eating disorder symptoms that need to be decreased, the coping strategies you could use some help with, and the self-care strategies that, frankly, you are pretty horrible with. We use this assessment to help us set goals to guide our approach to this program so take this exercise seriously. We don't DO ANYTHING YET. We are preparing and understanding (hence the name of the chapter).

PEP TALK TO SELF

> Ah yes, I am remembering now. I have actually been a pretty caring and thoughtful parent. This disorder has just thrown me off balance. And you know what? I am actually a pretty nice person. Stuff happens to everyone for a variety of reasons. If I had enough power to independently cause an eating disorder in my child, then I could cure it, right? I can only help him and guide his recovery. Therefore, I must not be the cause. Ah, I feel better. Thanks self, for the pep talk.

TIP BOX
Worry not. We will take each step bit by bit. You will not be doing anything you haven't done before; the disorder just makes it seem different. Now go back to your new, favorite corner, and have a few quiet moments.

Chapter TWO: Learning your approach and getting the family involved.

> I am really starting to enjoy this corner. In fact, I think my corner needs to be expanded into a room – or maybe a floor......

This section introduces you to our general approach for managing these disorders. This is our KEY SECTION. You learn about Off the C.U.F.F. You learn some tricks for eating disorder management. This is an important section. After reading this section, you are almost ready to go. However, you have one thing left to do before you jump in: THE FAMILY MEETING. Oh, we'll explain, just hold on.

The key to managing these disorders is working as a family to beat the disorder – not working against your child with the disorder. To this end, we suggest that you have a family planning meeting. The purpose of the meeting is to introduce your child to what changes he/she can expect from you, your willingness and ability to help him/her through this, and to gather his/her input on the most helpful way to proceed. A talk may go something like this:

"Daughter (Son) we need to have a chat. We (I) have been watching your health slowly deteriorate. Because I love you dearly, I cannot sit by and watch this continue. Thus, things have to change. I am here to help you get beyond this eating disorder that has taken you over. While your health is certainly not debatable, I want us to talk about the ways I can help you to fight this thing. For example, I can prepare all your meals for you and serve you, I can keep you company while you eat and afterwards, you can call me whenever you feel the urge to throw-up, etc.... "

TIP BOX

We usually tell parents their children are allowed to give input in the beginning to emphasize that this is a team effort. If your child's input is healthy and helps to fight the disorder, the input continues. However, if their disorder is too strong and their input only results in the disorder getting louder, than parents will take over more and more of the planning.

There are adaptations to these suggestions that we make according to your child's age and stage of the illness. These suggestions are found in the FREQUENTLY ASKED QUESTIONS section at the end of this chapter. However, it is important to note that many of the parents in our program have adult children. These skills work for all relationships and all situations. You'll see. It's all about understanding behavior. YEP. BACK TO YOUR NEW FAVORITE CORNER......JUST KEEP READING. We'll go through these stages one at a time.

WARNING: We start our weekly goals here.

Chapter THREE: Tricks to Implementing Your Approach.
In this section, we learn one of the most important skills in the entire program: the emotional wave. With this section, we start to get into a rhythm. We will set goals every week. The goals we set are based on our basic premise. Think of this as our code of honor, like the "golden rule" or something like that.

TIP BOX
Eating Disorders are coping strategies. Learning is a process.

A Word about Your Weekly Goals. To help your child, we will figure out how the disorder helps him or her to cope. We will work to INCREASE healthy coping skills. In the meantime, we will work to DECREASE unhealthy coping skills – a.k.a. eating disorder symptoms. How? We have found the best way for individuals to learn new skills is both to be taught how to do these skills and to have the skills demonstrated for them. Thus, we teach YOU how to do the things your children are not good at. In this manner, they can watch and learn from you! It is so much easier (and more enjoyable) when everyone is learning to do the same thing.

To do this, we set goals every week. We report on the progress or pitfalls of these goals at the beginning of every group. Goals relate to four major areas:
* Addressing an unhealthy or unhelpful behavior in your child.
* Targeting a healthy or helpful behavior in your child.
* Role modeling a healthy behavior yourself so your child can learn how to do it.
* Engaging in a SELF-CARE behavior for YOURSELF.

You will fill out a homework sheet each week. Depending on your therapy situation, you will use this sheet to check in with your therapist, your physician, your parent group, your web-based parent group, your social support......(the next chapter explains what we mean by social support). By now, I imagine the chair sees more of you than your significant other….

Chapter FOUR: Strengthening Your Team.
This is a brief section about making sure you have adequate support before you begin this program. We explain why this is so important and give you some suggestions if your circle of close confidents has gotten rather tiny. We also give you suggestions if you are having a tough time getting the other parent engaged in the process (if appropriate).

Chapter FIVE: Healthy Eating 101
We will teach you about the stages of nutrition when a child has a disorder. We will also examine what healthy eating means to you and your family. OK. Chair is not enough. Go on a date. If married, preferably with your spouse.

Chapter SIX: Understanding Behavior.
While we are setting goals and working to help your child manage this disorder, we are also going to be learning some helpful tools (or remembering tools that the disorder had temporarily caused us to forget). In this section, we help you remember how to change unhelpful behaviors in your children (and your friends) and replace them with helpful behaviors. Can you say "MASSAGE?"

Chapter SEVEN: Barriers to Behavior Change.
Ah, the best laid plans of mice and men....In this chapter, we highlight some common barriers to behavior change and help you to steer clear. I shouldn't even have to remind you of the chair by this point.

Chapter EIGHT: The Power of Example.
In this chapter, we help you ensure you are leading a lifestyle you wish for your child to emulate – one that balances work and leisure, one that favors learning and growing rather than outcomes.....

Chapter NINE: Process and You.
Physical Appearance, You, and Your Child. The symptoms of your child's illness necessitate that he or she devote a great deal of their mental resources to worrying about the way he or she looks. In order to help your child gain a healthy view of physical appearance (and start to walk proud and exude beauty), we have to take a look at our views of our own appearance and the value we place on it. It is hard not to get brain washed by all the media hype. We need to find our footing. Well, I didn't nag you last time. Did you do something anyway? (I am trying to give you more independence). Plans with friends would be nice.

Chapters TEN & ELEVEN: Creating a Healthy Meal Environment & The Joy of Eating
In this chapter, we hope to get you back to a healthy and mindful relationship to food. We discuss both the mental and physical aspects of the meal environment and address any discomforts you may have with food and eating. Can you say "FANCY RESTAURANT?"

Chapters TWELVE & THIRTEEN: Perfectionism.
Perfectionism. In this chapter, we help you understand the helpful and unhelpful aspects of perfectionism so you can help your children foster the healthy aspects and diminish the unhealthy aspects.

Chapters FOURTEEN & FIFTEEN: Emotion Regulation and Communication.
In these chapters, we highlight tools to help you understand your emotions so you can help your child regulate hers or his. We also address listening and communication. I shouldn't have to be nagging by this point.

Chapter SIXTEEN: The Journey of Recovery.
PARRR-TEEE!! By this point, you'll have a whole different perspective on life and recovery. Time to think about your path and prepare for the next phase of the journey.

Time for your first assignment. YEP, YOU GUESSED IT. BACK TO THE CHAIR.

TIP BOX

Remember, we go at YOUR pace. We take everything one step at a time. You choose the steps and you decide when to take the next one. We'll just help you figure out what steps to take and to not feel so alone while taking them.

Key Points

1   Life is a process. Focus on learning where you are rather than using so much energy worrying about where you have been and where you are going. It will help both you and your child to be more effective in the moment.

2   You can be most effective and helpful to your child if you role model healthy coping strategies and good self-parenting!

3   Your child's illness is a coping strategy, we need to teach your child better ways to cope.

4   Be patient with yourself. We learn with each step.

Weekly Goals

Your goal this week is information gathering. You are to take time to read the first two chapters and to observe how your family currently manages your child's eating disorder. Notice what is working and what is not working. This information will be vital for your first step: the family meeting.

Questions and Answers

Q: For what age child is this book written? My child is an adult who has been ill for a long time. This doesn't seem like it applies to me.

A: Never fear! The skills we teach in this program are important for good relationships. Period. Your approach with your child will depend on three factors:

1   Your child's age.
2   Your child's degree of financial independence (i.e. whether your child lives at home, is at college paid for by you, etc.).
3   The stage of your child's illness. We will help you modify your approach depending on these factors.

Q: Is the self-care really necessary? How many hours do you think I have in a week anyways?

A: I can't believe you asked me that. Sigh. We've got a lot of work to do with you, don't we? Yes, the self-care is ONE OF THE MOST IMPORTANT PARTS. Why? First, your child needs you. Taking care of yourself is essential so you don't burn out. Second, your child is not good at taking care of him or herself. Your child needs a role model of self-care and I pick YOU. Third, you're worth it. Life is short. Don't let it pass you by.

On that note…

My Gift to Myself This Week.

Find a private corner and a chair. Why am I harping on this so much? Well, it goes back to Virginia Wolfe's book <u>A Room of One's Own</u>. The premise of this important work is that everyone (in her time, women in particular) needs protected mental space. We need some area in which our time is protected; an escape place. A place where you assert a boundary, "OK everyone. I am going to my PLACE. I am not to be bothered for the next XX." You have to have this. You have to know that when you need to collect yourself, gather your thoughts, etc., you have a special place of peace. Some people have a tough time with transitions (e.g. coming home from work, etc.) For these people, this special place can help them ease into family life after a long day at work. I mean it. This is important.

CHAPTER ONE: Understanding your journey

Where You Are

✓ You have already finished your first step: you have learned more about the program.

Key Messages

It's a process: try, tweak, learn, grow.

Self-parenting is a necessary step for other-parenting.

Stay off the wave.

Remain genuine.

The Journey of Development

The purpose of this section is to give you an understanding of the nature of eating disorders, some thoughts about factors that contribute to eating disorder development, and an appreciation for our approach to managing these disorders. Eating disorders typically emerge at very pivotal periods of a child's development – such as adolescence. To understand why this may be, a helpful place to begin is to think about what healthy development looks like and to think about how eating disorders deviate from that.

Let's start with the goals of parenting. Basically, our job is to care for, love, and support our children so that they feel safe and can flourish; we then teach our children to care for, love, and support themselves. Our ultimate aim is for our children to function independently. As they mature and become adults, we want our children to come to us for guidance but do not rely on us for survival. If we were to simplify the tasks of parenting, these steps might look something like this.

Step One – Listen to their basic needs and provide for their basic needs

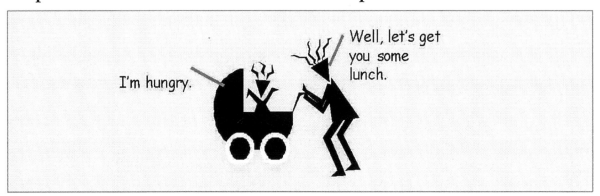

The child learns...

Hmmm…says the wise baby. When I am hungry, and I eat food, then I am no longer hungry and I feel satisfied and have energy. Eating is good for hunger and this person feeding me is pretty swell.

The Long Term Result of Step One

Your child learns how to listen to and to respect her/his hunger. S/he learns that hunger is nothing to be afraid of, but rather, hunger is a natural signal that our bodies give us to inform us that our bodies are in need of nourishment.

Step Two – Provide for their safety needs

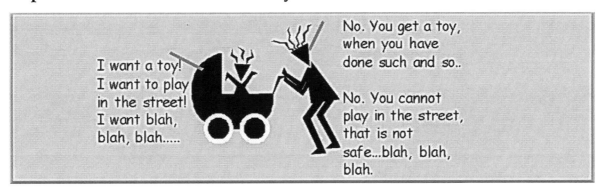

The child learns...

Aha! says the brilliant baby. You cannot always do everything you want. Sometimes your needs have to wait for an appropriate time; sometimes you are not ready to do certain things without certain skills.

The Long Term Result of Step Two

Your child learns about setting personal limits. Your child learns that you can't always do everything you want because there are costs and benefits associated with every decision. Your child learns how to make choices that maximize the positive consequences and minimize the negative consequences (much more on this later as difficulty with setting personal limits is a big problem for individuals with eating disorders).

Step Three – Provide for Their Emotional Needs

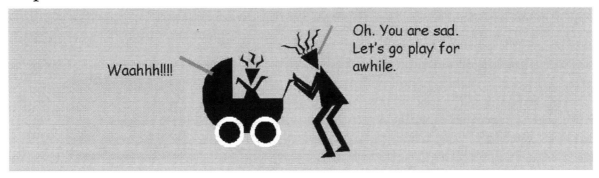

The child learns...

Oh!! says the genius baby. When I cry, that sometimes means I am sad. Being with others and doing fun things is what my sadness is telling me that I need.

The Long Term Result of Step Three

Your child learns not to fear her emotions. Rather, she learns that emotions give us information. Emotions may signal that she needs something, that something is wrong, or that everything is great. Your child learns to use this information to take care of herself, to respond to others, and to learn more about herself.

Step Four – Provide for their self-mastery needs

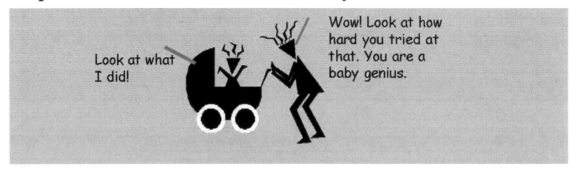

The child learns…

"Amazing!" says the child prodigy. "I can set goals and accomplish them. I am an amazing person."

The Long Term Result of Step Four

Your child learns to have confidence in his/her own ability to achieve goals. Your child learns that things don't always work out the way you want, but that you learn from everything you do so you can go about things differently the next time you try.

Step Five – Your child puts this all together, internalizes it, and learns to self-parent!

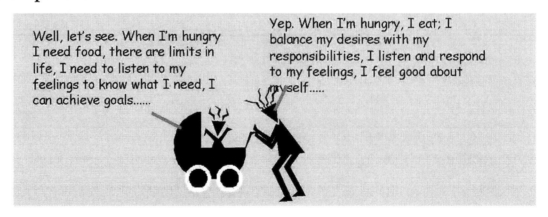

Ahh…sighs of a growing child.   I am ready to grow-up now.   I am figuring this whole thing out. I am learning how to listen to my body and respond to it. I am a swell self-parent.

The Long Term Result of Step Five

Your child learns to care for her/himself in a loving way both by how you have responded to her/his needs and by watching you care for YOURSELF.   In this manner, the messages your child receives are consistent.   Because what you do for yourself and your child match, your child gains trust that caring for oneself is a good idea. Your child has learned that our internal world (our energy level, our hunger, our feelings) give us messages and, by listening to these messages, we gain self-knowledge, self-trust, and confidence – the confidence of knowing that someone is always looking out for you: YOU!

Overwhelmed?

Don't be. What we are basically saying is this: Parenting is about three steps.

1. You provide for your child's needs by listening to and responding to your child (feeding hunger, validating emotions, setting limits). This is a messy process of trial and error, but that back and forth helps you to get to know your child better and for your child to trust you.
2. You teach your child to listen and respond to his or her own emotional and basic needs and to set limits. You do this by role modeling responding to your own needs, by teaching your children skills, by helping them set limits, and by role modeling balance.
3. As your child gets older, your child internalizes these lessons and takes on the task of listening to and responding to personal needs – i.e., they become self-parents!

Presto! A healthy child!

(Note: this rarely happens smoothly. It's the principle I'm trying to communicate)

Thus, in a perfect imaginary world, all of this goes smoothly and the end result of healthy parenting is that a child internalizes a kind and caring parent so that the child can self-parent. In other words, children learn to self-attune: to tune into the messages that their bodies send – of hunger, emotional experience, fatigue – etc, and respond to these needs in an adaptive way. By doing this back and forth dance with themselves, children get to know themselves, to trust themselves, and to feel safe within themselves. This security allows them to explore and discover what they are passionate about – and learn even more about themselves. Thus, by becoming a firm and warm self-parent, your children develop a sense of who they are and what they want.

It is perhaps not surprising to learn that this process does not seem to occur in individuals who develop an eating disorder. Rather than internalizing a kind and caring parent, having an eating disorder is like having a critical abusive parent inside your head. Individuals with eating disorders seem to ignore what their body is telling them (regarding feelings, hunger, fatigue, etc.). Instead, it is as if they have a rule book of how they think they "should be" or what they think others expect them to be and they just apply this rulebook to themselves no matter what their body is telling them.

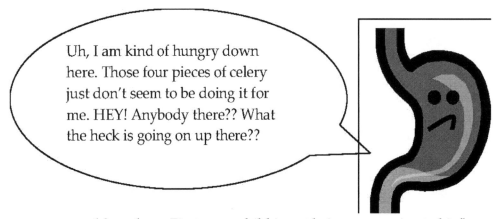

Uh, I am kind of hungry down here. Those four pieces of celery just don't seem to be doing it for me. HEY! Anybody there?? What the heck is going on up there??

There are two problems here. First, your child is not being responsive to his/her needs. Second, the rulebook he or she is applying is overly rigid, overly strict, overly restrictive, and frankly, cruel. To think why ignoring needs and applying unrealistic standards is not a good idea, think about the effect of a cruel insensitive parent on a young child (Note: this is NOT you. You are sitting here reading a book on how to help your child so don't let self-critical thoughts get in your way here. Just keep reading.).

Imagine this interchange occurring on a DAILY basis.

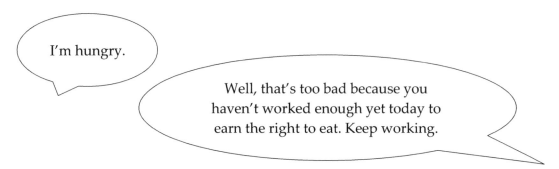

I'm hungry.

Well, that's too bad because you haven't worked enough yet today to earn the right to eat. Keep working.

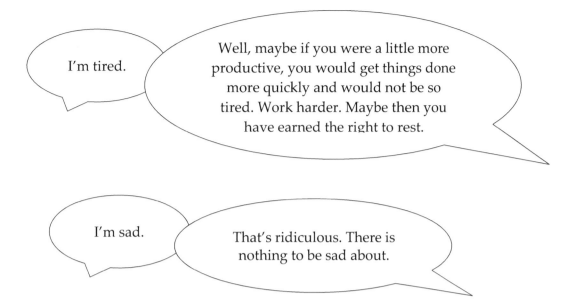

I'm tired.

Well, maybe if you were a little more productive, you would get things done more quickly and would not be so tired. Work harder. Maybe then you have earned the right to rest.

I'm sad.

That's ridiculous. There is nothing to be sad about.

So, does this child develop into a happy, confident child? Odds are against it. Sadly, this is likely the way your child motivates him or herself. Rather than kind guidance and reasonable limits, he or she pushes without listening to needs. The end result is that these children do not get to know themselves well or trust themselves. They just don't feel safe.

The Path to Disordered Eating

So why do certain children **not** internalize a warm and firm self-parent? Every time I treat a new family, they always ask, "Why did my child get an eating disorder?" I figured I may as well just get this question out of the way.

THE ANSWER: There are no easy answers. One thing we know for sure. There is never "one cause" for an eating disorder. Life is just not that simple. Let's face it. Eating disorders have been around for hundreds of years. If the answer were simple, wouldn't we have figured it out by now? This being said, we do know a few things. We summarize what we know here (with broad strokes, it would take a whole book to get into the weeds on this).

✿ Perfectionist's Corner ✿

<u>Perfectionist</u>:   But I want answers. How can I stop feeling guilty if someone doesn't tell me it is not my fault?

<u>Voice of Reason</u>:   It is not your fault. You didn't wake up one day and say "Today is the day I give my child an eating disorder." You did not get your child here. You just do not have that kind of power. However, your child does need you to help her get out of this. To be of the most help to your child, trust that you have always done what you believed to be best for your child. You have. With your heart in the right place and your determination set, you and your family will conquer this disorder.

Factors that Contribute to Disordered Eating

The study of risk factors - biological, social, psychological, etc… features of an individual that increase the likelihood that they will develop a disorder, has been very challenging and largely inconclusive. Yet, despite that, we can describe individuals with anorexia nervosa relatively precisely. We just aren't sure where it came from.

On the one hand, they appear to be very driven individuals. This is called many things, including perfectionism (we spend a few chapters on this later in the program). In brief, this means they often set untenably high demands or standards for their bodies and their performance. Being driven may or may not be a problem in itself. There is actually some debate on this. However, when this drive is combined with two things: trouble learning from experience and a punitive attitude towards oneself when things don't go well, that's when problems can start.

In other words, individuals with eating disorders are very hard on themselves when they feel they do not meet their driven standards and don't seem particularly good at learning to do things differently the next time. Some other complications: they are extremely sensitive to the negative evaluations of others, and they tend to avoid situations in which there is uncertainty in how to behave (e.g., unstructured time with classmates) or in which the standards for rating performance are ambiguous. These latter factors may make the consequences of mistakes particularly punitive and the opportunities to practice more limited.

In terms of their intrapersonal experience (or self-parenting), as we have noted, they are not very good at attuning: at changing their behavior or goals in response to what their bodies are telling them. On the one hand, they tend to be extremely sensitive to how their body feels. For example, they often have gastrointestinal and other somatic symptoms that far predate the beginning of their eating disorder – one sign of this sensitivity to bodily experience. Now, here is something that can be tricky to understand. Individuals also feel emotions in their bodies. We get a knot in our gut when we will guilty, we get butterflies when we feel anxious – and so on. Thus, one line of thinking is that individuals who are more sensitive to how their body feels experience stronger emotions. Thus, one way of thinking of individuals with anorexia nervosa (and potentially other eating disorders) is they experience life with a BANG! and a POW!: the world is an intense, vivid experience and they are emotional sponges who soak it all up: individuals who are extremely sensitive to the world around them and to their own internal experience. This is gift, as they are passionate creatures, but it can be a lot to handle sometimes.

However, one key to anorexia nervosa (and potentially other eating disorders) is understanding how they respond to what they sense. Critically, they do not use the information that their body gives them to guide their decisions and their behavior. As a result, they do not develop the self-trust and self-knowledge that comes from regularly tuning into yourself and learning about what you like and need.

WHY?? Well, we don't know. The unsatisfying but most reasonable answer is their biology combined with life experiences and crappy timing. For example, one possibility is that your driven child was probably rewarded for such excessive hard work that resulted in ignoring needs and setting unhealthy limits. Coaches love children who work really hard. Teachers love children who work really hard. Other parents admire you for having a child who works so hard. Other children admire children who get such positive accolades. Over time, the driven behavior and poor self-parenting get rewarded – although there are so many, many, paths to these outcomes.

Wait just a minute here. Why is this strategy bad if it is so successful? I know my child is happy when he or she is successful and I want my child to be happy.

A Confused but Well-Intentioned Parent

Parenting a driven child is very tricky indeed. What we have to ask ourselves is NOT how well they are achieving goals, but rather at WHAT COST? Are tangible measures of success (good grades, athletic awards, etc.) truly "success" if they are earned while sacrificing one's physical health, mental health, self-trust, inner peace, and self-knowledge? (that was rhetorical). Just because one's methods for achieving a certain goal worked, does not mean that there aren't alternative methods that are MORE effective with less COST. It just takes a certain degree of courage to try a new method.

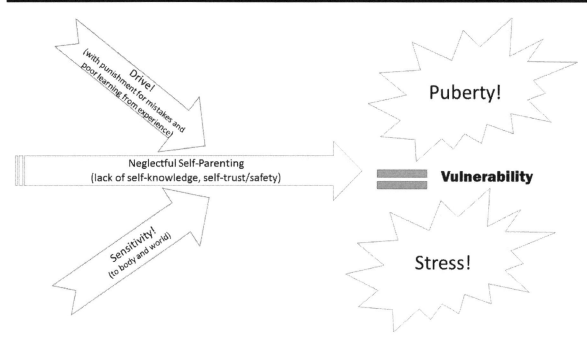

Figure 1

Notwithstanding all of this, while these features may increase the likelihood, the presence of these characteristics **does not guarantee that an eating disorder will develop.** There are many, many people who have these features but don't have an eating disorder.

Eating disorders may be more likely to develop during times of stress. Thus, it is helpful to think of eating disorders as a way of coping with things. Often it is not ONE big stressor that sets the stage, but rather a series of smaller stressors that may increase the likelihood. We will explain why eating disorders work so well to help your child cope on the following pages. See Figure One for a a visual summary of all the things we just talked about.

Now, just because we can't say what caused the eating disorder doesn't mean that we don't know how to treat it and how to prevent it from returning.

We are extremely confident in the following things that we do know:

Your child is not good at caring for herself/himself.

You are essential for your child's recovery.   You can really help your child through this time.

Your job:

To care for your child.

To teach your child to care for herself or himself.

How?   Well, that's what this program is all about.

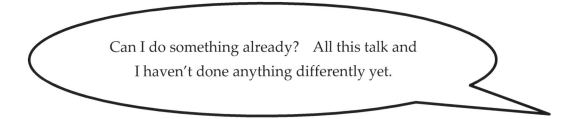

Role modeling ignoring.......

How Does an Eating Disorder Help a Child Cope with Things?

Consider a theory of motivation developed by a psychologist named Abraham Maslow. He developed a theory to help explain what motivates people to do what they do.   ]This theory is often known as the "hierarchy of needs." He proposed that our needs are arranged in order of necessity. He felt that until individuals have satisfied lower level needs, higher level needs will not and cannot be sought. An outline of this theory is below.

As you can see, people with eating disorders are stuck at the bottom level. They have an internalized a cruel, insensitive parent (their eating disorder) which prevents them from meeting their most basic need: feeding their hunger. Because of this, over time individuals with eating disorders certainly do not feel safe (level 2). How could anyone feel safe who is not being fed and cared for properly?!!! Over time, what happens is that your child loses interest in (or at least contact with) all the higher levels. They may lose interest in friends, activities, etc. This is actually is one way of thinking about how the eating disorder acts as a coping strategy: by being stuck on the first level, your child's world becomes narrowly focused on food and all the other worries fade into background! Thus, in some ways, the eating disorder simplifies life for your child. As you will come to learn through this program, our job is to take your child through these levels of development.

To apply these concepts to your child and your family, let's walk together through the symptoms your child is experiencing along with the coping strategies s/he is not very skilled at practicing. We may then have a better idea of how the eating disorder helps your child cope.

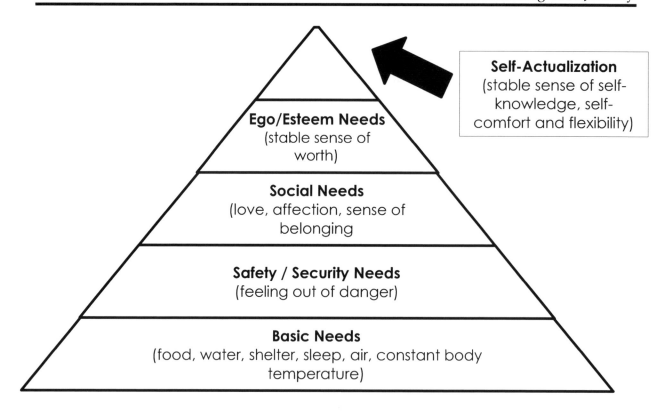

For this to make sense, don't forget these key points. This serves as the reasoning behind our entire intervention.

TIP BOX
Key Points of the Program – remember these

1. You can think of eating disorders as coping strategies. In order for an individual to want to give up a coping strategy, we have to teach him or her more effective ways to cope.

2. The best way for someone to learn a coping strategy is not only to be given information, but also for important people (you) to practice the coping strategy as well (HMMM). This shows your child how important this skill really is.

3. One skill your child is not good at is doing nice, kind things for him/herself. SOOO, each week you will do nice things for yourself. This not only helps you to PREVENT burnout, but also shows your child that we all deserve to be cared for. Yep, you're worth it. JUST BECAUSE.

Overwhelmed? Well, worry not. We will guide you through, RIGHT NOW, to think about what we just taught you in terms of your child and yourself. We want you to think carefully about the following questions and to WRITE DOWN YOUR ANSWERS. Writing things down is a powerful strategy, in and of itself, because it makes you more aware of things you may not have noticed. Things look a lot different on paper than when they are floating around in your head. Here are a few tips:

1) Keep things very specific and small.
2) Think behaviors: things you and your child can DO.
3) You may need to think where they are now, where you want them to be, and think what the first baby step towards that goal would be…

Family Assessment: Questions about You and Your Child

Step One: **What are some of the UNHEALTHY and UNHELPFUL behaviors of my child?**   These include eating disorder behaviors, behaviors that interfere with family relationships, and anything else you think interferes with your child's functioning.

Write what your child needs to work on here.

- doesn't eat enough food
- doesn't ~~to~~ enjoy eating → eating is stressful
- eats limited "safe" foods
- "safe" food list is diminishing.
- constantly thinks about food + exercise
- very sad/hopeless/"dreads the day"
- bad mood all the time
- very non-communicative

Suggestion Box

Doesn't eat enough food
Throws up after meals
Takes diet pills
Eats a limited variety of foods (no fat, no desserts, no protein)
Only eats sandwiches on odd days of the month
Exercises too much
Has inappropriate use of condiments or artificial sweetener
Consumes excessive diet drinks
Takes two years to complete a meal

Step Two: **What are some helpful coping strategies my child would benefit from improving?**   Parents sometimes have a tough time identifying the things their children struggle to cope with because their children are not good at identifying this themselves. To help you with this, I give you the unhelpful skill and the healthy alternative in the Suggestion Box on the next page. I hope this helps.

Write what your child needs to work on here.

- Not good at expressing feelings effectively
- Not good at saying no
- Has trouble understanding the middle way. Sees everything in black + white
- Not good at resolving conflict - tends to get and stay angry @ people or tolerating someone who is mad at her.
- Has trouble doing nice things for herself. Trouble balancing leisure time + work.

Suggestion Box	
Unhelpful Behavior **(what you may see)**	**Healthy Behavior** **(what we will be working on to improve)**
Not good at asking for help. Always puts on a happy face, never comes to friends or family with problems.	Being honest with self and others when s/he is struggling and asks for help. Does not feel guilty asking for help. (Chapter 4)
Not good at coping with mistakes. Criticizes him or herself or feels very guilty or shameful with even minor mistakes. Sometimes this shows itself as never admitting they are wrong.	Views mistakes as opportunities for learning. (Chapter 2 and on)
Not good at expressing feelings effectively. Either you see extreme outbursts of intense emotions or all the emotions are kept in and you rarely see them.	Expresses feelings effectively. (All through the book)
Not good at setting limits for her or himself. Takes on too many activities, studies way too long and sacrifices sleep; helps friends beyond reason.	Pays attention to inner feedback and uses that feedback to guide limits (Chapters 7,8,9)
This is important. Parents often overlook this one because it seems like their child can "handle it." However, when you look closely, you realize this is at great personal expense: they do it at the expense of their health and happiness.	
Not good at saying no. You see them doing things you know they would rather not do…volunteering for things they don't have time for).	Considers desires and personal needs and says "no" when necessary (and watches the negative thoughts that come out of habit go by (Chapters 7,8,9)
Has trouble understanding the middle way. Sees everything in black and white: people are good or bad; a test is failed or perfect, etc.	Views life as an experience and opportunity for learning.
Not good at resolving conflict. Tends to get and STAY angry with others or has a great deal of trouble tolerating when others are mad at her/him.	Accepts that others make mistakes and works to have reasonable expectations.
Has trouble doing nice things for him or herself. Has trouble balancing leisure time and work.	Does a lovely, nice thing for her or himself every day. *Carpe Diem, baby!*

Step Three: Helpful Coping Strategies <u>I Need to Work on</u> for Role Modeling

Refer to the Suggestion Box below.

Write what you would benefit from working on here.

Suggestion Box	
Unhelpful Behavior **(what you may see)**	**Healthy Alternative** **(that we will work on increasing)**
You are not good at asking for help. Always put on a happy face, never comes to friends or family with problems.	You are honest with yourself and others when you are struggling and ask for help! And learn that any guilt you feel for asking for help is misplaced.
You are not good at coping with mistakes. You criticize yourself or feel guilty or shameful for mistakes. As a result, you may have trouble acknowledging mistakes.	You view mistakes as opportunities for learning.
You are not good at expressing feelings effectively. You keep your feelings inside until your explode; you explode all the time or you keep everything in.	You express feelings effectively.
You are not good at setting limits for yourself (you take on too many activities, **DO TOO MANY THINGS FOR YOUR CHILD(REN),** work too long and sacrifice sleep, and /or help friends and children beyond reason.	You pay attention to inner feedback and use that feedback to guide limits.
You are not good at saying no or setting limits on your children for fear you will upset them, they will be upset or disappointed with you, etc.	You consider desires and personal needs and say "no" when necessary and watch the negative thoughts that come out of habit go by.
You have trouble understanding the middle way. Sees everything in black and white: people are good or bad; the house is perfect or filthy, at project at work is a victory or failure, etc.	You view life as an experience and opportunity for learning.

Suggestion Box	
Unhelpful Behavior **(what you may see)**	**Healthy Alternative** **(that we will work on increasing)**
You are not good at resolving conflict. You tend to get and STAY angry with others or have difficulty tolerating when others are angry with you.	You accept people, including yourself, making mistakes and work to have reasonable expectations of yourself and others.
You place unrealistic demands on yourself. You have trouble balancing leisure time and work.	You do a lovely, nice thing for yourself every day. *Carpe Diem, baby!*
You don't take good physical care of yourself. You don't eat, exercise and sleep properly.	You eat, exercise, rest and balance in a healthy way.
You have trouble apologizing. You always apologize with a "Sorry, BUT…"	You say, "I'm sorry" and STOP.
You have trouble complimenting without teaching. "That's great, BUT…"	You applaud and STOP.

Step Four: What are the self-care behaviors that I could use work on?

Write your 'need to work on' here.
· new hobbies
· time w/ keith
· need to take pride in my physical appearance
· need to have more respect for myself in general

Suggestion Box

Don't make regular mealtimes a priority

Sacrifice my sleep for others

Need to learn a new hobby

Need to spend time ALONE with my spouse

Need to set a regular time I stop work each day

Need to take weekends off

Need to buy something for myself

Need to exercise in a MODERATE manner

Need to take pride in my physical appearance

Need to have more respect for myself in general.   I am a decent person after

Oh stop it! I can just feel you worrying about this. No worries. We use these goals to guide the WHOLE PROGRAM. We will use this sheet as a guide that will help you design your homework assignments each week. Each week, our homework will contain four parts.

1. Each week we will focus on an unhealthy or unhelpful behavior in your child (this is one of the unhealthy behaviors that you listed in Step One).

2. We will then work on improving a healthy behavior in your child (these are the behaviors that your child needs to work on that you listed in Step Two).

3. We will work on role modeling a healthy coping strategy for YOURSELF. (these are the things you listed in Step Three).

4. Finally, you will set a self-care goal so that we can make sure you are taking care of yourself during this process and role modeling how important this is. For now, just trust us that this is VERY IMPORTANT. We go into the details of 'why' later.

The homework sheet that you will fill out each week is found at the end of this section. In your weekly goals, we will tell you how to use it for your first assignment.

Key Points

Let's summarize what we have learned about parenting and eating disorders. In the next section, we'll explain what the experience of an eating disorder is like for your child and how an "Off the C.U.F.F." approach can make it easier for both you and your child to manage the disorder.

1. The main goal of parenting is for your child to learn to be a kind and supportive parent for him or herself.

2. Children with eating disorder have yet to internalize this parent. Instead they have internalized a cruel, unforgiving parent, an eating disorder.

3. Their eating disorder serves as a coping strategy. We need to figure out how their disorder helps them cope so we can teach them healthier strategies. You have already done this ☺.

4. Talk is cheap. The best way for your children to learn healthy strategies is for you to role model them (it's good for you too.)

5. Taking care of your self is an extremely important part of this program. It communicates to your child that this is important, is shows your child how to do it, and you are worth it!

Weekly Goals

We start off easy. Your first goal is to ONLY FILL OUT #4 on your homework page. Yep, your only job this week is doing something nice for yourself.

Questions and Answers

Q: Don't you think it's time we started working on my child's disorder now?
A: Why yes, you anticipated me. With your obvious eagerness, and your soon-to-be-superior self-care, we are ready. Read on. The next few sections are key.

Q: I have several children. How can I involve my spouse when someone has to care for the children?
A: An eating disorder is a family problem. As a family, it is important to discuss what is going on with your child and how everyone can support your child in getting help. It is important that both you and your spouse (or the child's other parent) read this book and set weekly goals. It is VERY IMPORTANT that you support each other in the goals you set. As far as involving the children, when one family member is in trouble, the family needs to work together to make sure the person with the disorder is supported in health, but the disorder does not run the family. We'll explain this more in the next section. In brief, the family supports behaviors towards health in all of its members but does not support behaviors that prolong illness. Treatment is good, so the family mobilizes to make sure treatment can happen. It is best if both parents can come if you are part of a treatment group, however, if this is not possible, have one parent be the index person and the other parent come AS OFTEN AS POSSIBLE – this communicates an important message to your child.

Q: I am a very private person. I am just not comfortable talking to others about my problems.
A: Thanks for being honest about your struggles. When you go to your chair after reading this, I want you to think about the barriers that make it hard for you to share. Maybe you have been taught that asking for help is a sign of weakness? Maybe you don't want to burden others with your struggle? Think for a moment how you feel when someone comes to you with their troubles and asks you for support or advice. Makes you feel important and trusted, doesn't it? Asking for help is a balancing act, a dance between people. We have to balance meeting our own needs with asking. It is not our job to anticipate or mind-read how much help is appropriate. Rather, it is the job of other peoples to communicate their personal boundaries so we know when we are asking for too much.

Wisdom of the Week: My Gift to Myself

Think of a mistake you made this week and focus on what you learned from it.   If you criticized yourself for it, apologize to yourself for being such a jerk and know that, although criticizing yourself may be a habit, that doesn't mean you have to believe it because, frankly, it is not true. This can be especially important to remember when you're going through a stressful time, like supporting a family member who has an eating disorder.

GOALS FOR WEEK #1

Date:

Remember our key guidelines
It's a process! Try, tweak, grow and learn.
Self-parenting: a necessary prerequisite for other parenting.
Learn how to SURF The WAVE!
Remain genuine.

Eats too little	Eats too little variety	Exercises too much
Throws up after meals	Doesn't get enough sleep	Doesn't set limits
Abuses laxatives	Engages in self-harm	Other

Possible Suggestions of How to Address:	**My Plan:**
☐ Ignore it ☐ Have a discussion about needed change in behavior *(discuss a future, necessary, logical consequence given the severity of the behavior)* ☐ Implement a logical consequence (reminding your child of the importance of health before anything) ☐ Appeal to your child's inner wisdom (have a discussion with your child about what you have observed, why you are concerned, the change in behavior expected) ☐ Reverse Time-Out (you leave) ☐ Group Time-Out (everyone leaves for 10 minutes) ☐ Regrouping (family meeting to get out of power struggle) ☐ Humor	Would a discussion be a good idea?

Heathy Coping Strategy I will address with my child this week and my plan to address it.

Expressing negative emotions effectively	Asking for help	Setting limits (studies too much, too many activities)
Expressing opinions	Being considerate of others	Placing realistic demands on self (consider the cost, not whether she achieves them)
Better balance of work and leisure	Increasing grey vs black & white thinking	Managing disappointing results
Increasing confidence in appearance	Increasing confidence in intellect	Other

Possible Suggestions:	**My Plan:**
☐ Positive attention when takes a step towards Behavior ☐ One-on-one time outside of eating disorder stuff ☐ Earning a logical privilege given increased health ☐ Praise and STOP – no BUTS ☐ Role Model Behavior Yourself ☐ Open the door for a discussion ☐ Set a limit ☐ Offer to teach ☐ Other	

Heathy Coping Strategy I will Role Model this week.	
Possible Suggestions:	**My Plan:**
☐ Delegate something.	
☐ Say 'no' to some things.	
☐ Be honest with my feelings.	
☐ Express my feelings when not on the wave.	
☐ Ask for help.	
☐ Set healthy limits between my needs and those of others.	
☐ Listen with full attention.	
☐ Praise and STOP.	
☐ Say "I'm sorry" with no excuses.	
☐ Allow family members to make mistakes without jumping in.	
☐ Be consistent.	
☐ Address negative self-talk.	
☐ Be reliable.	

Self-care Strategy I will implement this week	
Possible Suggestions:	**My Plan:**
☐ Make regular mealtimes a priority.	
☐ Set a regular bedtime.	
☐ Learn a new hobby.	
☒ Spend some time with my friends.	· Bonfire @ A's
☐ Spend time ALONE with my spouse.	
☐ Set a regular time I stop work each day.	
☐ Take weekends off.	No lame excuses!!
☐ Buy something for myself.	
☐ Exercise in a MODERATE manner.	
☒ Take pride in my physical appearance.	· reduce body shaming

TIP OF THE WEEK: BE YOUR OWN CARING PARENT

CHAPTER TWO: Learning Your Approach

Where You Are

- ✓ You have finished your first step.   You have learned more about the program.

- ✓ You have learned more about the stages of parenting and how eating disorders take your child off the path of healthy growth.

Congratulations.

Topic: Off the C.U.F.F.

This section introduces you to our general approach for managing eating disorders. This is our KEY SECTION. You learn about Off the C.U.F.F. You learn some tricks for eating disorder management. After reading this section, believe it or not, we start making some serious changes in the family.

> I am really starting to enjoy this corner.   In fact, I think my corner needs to be expanded into a room

Let's combine what we have learned about healthy development with what we know about eating disorders. From this, our approach to parenting and disorder management will make a lot of sense (I am hoping).

Remember: the end result of healthy child development is that your child internalizes a kind and caring parent who uses positive discipline rather than critical punishment to set limits and achieve goals. Well, rather than internalizing a kind and caring parent, having an eating disorder is like having a cruel, neglectful, and evil parent inside your head. The eating disorder tells your child to ignore her/his hunger. The eating disorder doesn't care if your child is tired and will tell him/her to keep working anyway. The eating disorder hates feelings so it does not bother to listen to the feelings of your child but tells him/her to ignore them (or express them in a powerful way). The eating disorder insults your child as a way to motivate her/him to try harder, and very importantly, THE EATING DISORDER IS NEVER SATISFIED.

It is helpful to think of my trick to understanding what an eating disorder is like inside of his or her head.

Secret Trick to Understanding Eating Disorders:
AN EATING DISORDER IS LIKE A TEMPER TANTRUM.

If you understand this, you can understand how an eating disorder thinks.

Let's consider this carefully. Think back to when your young children had temper tantrums because they wanted something. That didn't take long.

What do we know about tantrums? Simply:

- if the tantrum worked to get the child what he or she wanted, expect a tantrum the next time he or she doesn't get what s/he wants.

- if the tantrum didn't work, than it is less likely you'll see it again (but your child will test you several times before s/he makes this conclusion AND FIRST IT MAY GET WORSE BEFORE IT GETS BETTER).

- If your child is punished after having a tantrum, you guessed it, less likely the next time.

- If your child is complimented when s/he doesn't have a tantrum, yep, less likely,

BUT, here is the trickiest part...if the tantrums work SOME of the time it will take a lot longer for them to go away.   In fact, if you had been giving in to tantrums and then decide "nah, this is not a good idea" – they'll get worse before they get better. Why? Well, because they worked before for goodness sakes! Your child is not going to give up that easy!   First s/he will make them stronger to see if that does the trick.

The Clever, but Devious, Child

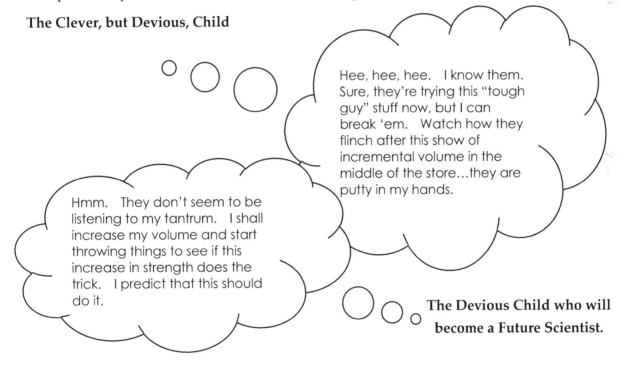

Hee, hee, hee.   I know them. Sure, they're trying this "tough guy" stuff now, but I can break 'em.   Watch how they flinch after this show of incremental volume in the middle of the store...they are putty in my hands.

Hmm.   They don't seem to be listening to my tantrum.   I shall increase my volume and start throwing things to see if this increase in strength does the trick.   I predict that this should do it.

The Devious Child who will become a Future Scientist.

Hey, don't blame me. You did the same thing when you were a child. In fact, temper tantrums follow the basic rules of all behavior. These are important (so we put them in a box). Actually, understanding these rules will help you for the rest of your life. These rules will not only help you with the eating disorder, but they will help you with any behavior that you are trying to change in your child, your spouse, your elderly parent, your dog.

> **TIP BOX**
>
> **Laws of Behavior (Why everyone does what to do)**
>
> Rule #1   Behaviors increase when the behavior is followed by something that we like.
> Example: Every time I make my bed, my dad gives me a dollar.   If I like money, I will make sure I make my bed on a daily basis.
>
> Rule #2   Behaviors increase when the behavior ends something that we don't like.
> Example: My sister is always nagging and insulting me.   When I kick her, she stops. I will increase my kicking whenever she nags me. True story.
>
> Rule #3   Behaviors decrease when they result in things that we don't like.
> Example: If every time I behave disrespectfully to my mom, I lose the car keys for the next day.   Eventually I will get the connection and will decrease insulting my mom.

O.K. Back to temper tantrums. We can apply those rules to get rid of temper tantrums. Since your child's eating disorder acts like a tantrum inside her head, these rules can help us to manage her eating disorder!

HOW DO YOU GET RID OF A TEMPER TANTRUM?

SHORT ANSWER: You ignore it – EVERYTIME IT HAPPENS.   Why? Because then the behavior doesn't work for your child to get what s/he wants.

LONG ANSWER: You use principles of behavior management (the three rules) to understand the function of the tantrum (why your child doing it) and you teach your child a better way to get his or her needs met.

The Eating Disorder as a Temper Tantrum

Why do I think an eating disorder acts like a temper tantrum in your child's head? Well, let's visit your child at lunch, and I'll explain why.

First, let's meet, Egor, your child's eating disorder. At every meal, Egor throws a little fit inside your child's head in an effort to get your child to eat less food. Why? Well, Egor's goal is to have your child lose more and more weight so your child becomes more and more isolated, robotic, and rigid, and Egor gains more power.

**This is the eating disorder.
We'll call it EGOR.**

How does Egor attempt to do this? Well, Egor is not the most sophisticated of creatures and uses very childlike strategies. It has a tantrum inside your child's head. It calls your child names. It threatens all these unrealistic consequences that have no basis in reality.

A Temper Tantrum: The Taunts and Threats	An Eating Disorder: The Taunts and Threats
"If you don't buy me that toy, I won't have any friends. All the other kids have that toy and no one will like me if I don't have it. Besides, I am going to scream and I am not going to love you anymore if you don't buy it for me."	"If you eat that, you'll never be able to stop eating and you'll get fatter and fatter."

"You must do everything you can to avoid eating. If you don't try to hide food, you are not trying hard enough and that will show how lazy you are."

"Don't trust these people. They are just jealous and just want to get you fat. Only I know best. If you don't listen to me, you'll be sorry and I will make you feel very, very guilty."

"I can feel your thighs growing by the second. That piece of celery is going right to your hips."

"Don't walk past that bakery. The smell may put you under."

"You know of you start eating good tasting food, you won't be able to shop." |

Let's think about our temper tantrum analogy and think of your child's different options in responding to Egor.

♦ If your child gives in to Egor (does what it says), Egor shuts up for a little while and your child experiences less guilt in that moment (just like you would experience temporary calm if you give in to your child's tantrum).

That moment feels good. It is similar to how one would feel if one got an 'A' on an assignment in the class of an overly critical and demanding teacher.

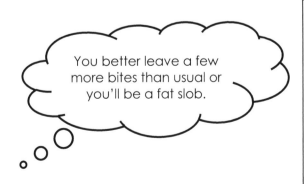

Option 1: Eat less, satisfy Egor and have temporary peace (think temper tantrum after long day at work – you get the picture!)

Option 2: Ignore and have to endure Egor getting louder and more insistent in the short term (increased intensity of tantrum in store when you initially say no).

♦ If your child ignores Egor, there is a short term penalty: Egor will get a lot louder before it gets quieter. Why? Well, when something that has worked does not work, we usually try harder before we give up. (We'll learn more about this in later chapters but think of how your child's tantrum would get louder in a store if you weren't listening...at first).

♦ It's what happens at the next few meals that are important. If Egor won the last time (i.e. your child gave in), it will be back – but it will want MORE at the next meal (human nature: we always push for more). This is the downward spiral we see in eating disorders. At each meal, Egor tries to get your child to eat less and less...if it won the last time.

♦ If your child ignored Egor, distracted him or herself from Egor's taunts, held your hand, sat with you for support or did whatever he or she needed to do to ignore Egor, Egor will certainly try again every meal for at least the next few days (it won't give up that easy). But if you and your child develop a good support system for ignoring, it will start to get quieter...just like if you ignored your *child's* tantrums three stores in a row, by the fourth store...

**Eating Disorder
Disillusionment**

I don't understand what is going on here! Am I getting old? Past my prime? Are my threats outdated? Clearly, I need to move to a new host...

Make sense? Then, we're almost ready. Let's think how using an Off the C.U.F.F. style can help you help your child with his or her eating disorder. It is the style we have found works best in giving your child confidence that you and s/he can take on this disorder!

> **TIP BOX**
>
> We have found that an Off the C.U.F.F. approach is a great "style" to use for disorder management and for parenting in general!

Off the C.U.F.F.

Off the C.U.F.F. is a style of parenting – a style of communicating, establishing rules and guidelines, and teaching children we have found to be very effective. Why "Off the C.U.F.F.?" Here is why.

C is for Clear. C is our big "Communication" letter. Communication is vital for effective parenting. Often both parent and child do not clarify their expectations but think instead "Oh, he or she must know what I mean by that."

Take a simple example – room cleaning.

Parent says to child, "Clean your room."

To the parent, this means:

> Surely, my obedient child knows "clean your room" means stop everything right now; go upstairs immediately; dust, vacuum, put away clean clothes; get everything put away and off the floor.

However, to the child this means:

> Before I leave home to go to college in a few years, I need to shove all my things under the bed.

You know what I'm talking about. In all likelihood, this has happened to you before. Now, in terms of dealing with the Eating Disorder, instead of, "Make sure you eat lunch," you say, "OK. We have to increase lunches to include a sandwich, chips and milk. You have told me you can do this on your own, but I haven't seen any change, so it appears that you need more support. I am going to fix it for you and keep you company while you eat to help you. When you can do it on your own, I'll step back." Clear? You bet.

TAKE HOME POINT – ASSUME NOTHING

   ✓ Be clear about what you expect from your children and be clear what your expectations are regarding the management of your child's disorder.

U is for Undisturbed. A parent remaining undisturbed (calm, confident, etc.) is extremely important. This communicates several things to your child. It communicates:
   o You know what you are doing.

o   You can handle this situation.

o   This situation is no big deal and nothing to worry about.

Your child looks to you for guidance and as a strong source of support.   Not feeling it?
Fake it until you make it, baby.   We'll help.   The confidence will come, but your child
needs you to be strong now to get through this. If you are undisturbed, it gives your
child the message that managing the disorder is possible, that you know exactly what
needs to be done.

To illustrate what I mean, think about the difference between the ANXIOUS PARENT
and the UNDISTURBED PARENT.

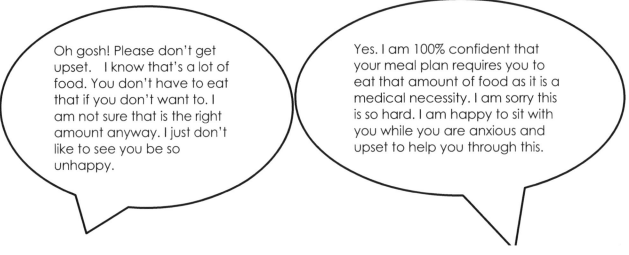

Oh gosh! Please don't get upset.   I know that's a lot of food. You don't have to eat that if you don't want to. I am not sure that is the right amount anyway. I just don't like to see you be so unhappy.

Yes. I am 100% confident that your meal plan requires you to eat that amount of food as it is a medical necessity. I am sorry this is so hard. I am happy to sit with you while you are anxious and upset to help you through this.

The Anxious Parent

The Undisturbed Parent

TAKE HOME POINT – STAY CALM AND CLEAR.

✓   If you are calm and clear, it increases your child's confidence that what you are
saying is the appropriate thing to do.

Undisturbed is important for another reason as well.   We don't want the disorder to
take control of your family.   We want parents to remain at the helm and children
having more and more input as they age (and grow wiser?).   When the Eating Disorder
causes us to lose our cool (i.e. we get angry), the disorder is quite happy.   Why?   It
knows it is getting to you and getting more powerful.

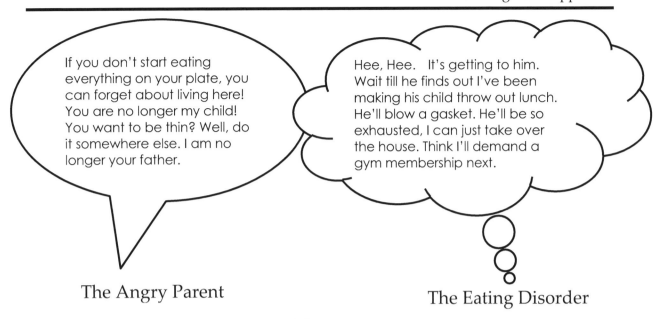

If you don't start eating everything on your plate, you can forget about living here! You are no longer my child! You want to be thin? Well, do it somewhere else. I am no longer your father.

The Angry Parent

Hee, Hee. It's getting to him. Wait till he finds out I've been making his child throw out lunch. He'll blow a gasket. He'll be so exhausted, I can just take over the house. Think I'll demand a gym membership next.

The Eating Disorder

TAKE HOME POINT – KEEP YOUR COOL.

✓ Losing your cool gives the eating disorder power because it knows it can influence you. When you remain undisturbed, you don't reinforce the disorder with attention or power. Stay cool.

TIP BOX

Remember that special, quiet place I made you create in the last chapter? Well, here is where it really comes into use. When you find yourself getting agitated or frustrated, excuse yourself gracefully, say you'll return after you clear your head, and go spend some time there. As long as you need (much more on this in the next chapter).

F is for Firm. By "firm" we refer to the manner in which you communicate expectations. We don't need to be firm all the time, certainly, only when it appears that things are getting a little out of hand. Why? Your child should know you are confident about what needs to happen as a firm tone makes your child feel less anxious.

This is the point at which I often get protests from parents of older children who find that being firm has outlived its usefulness. Yes and no. Let's think this through. Certain things are not negotiable – no matter what the age your child is.

Furthermore, when it comes to eating disorders, we need to get away from thoughts of **CHRONOLOGICAL AGE** (how many years they have lived) and think about **DEVELOPMENTAL AGE** (what developmental tasks they have achieved). Time for a tip box.

TIP BOX

Think of your child in terms of developmental age (what stages of development he or she has achieved) rather than how old he or she is.

Young children can rest when they are tired, eat when they are hungry, etc. If you child struggles with this, her or his developmental is much younger than her or his chronological age.

Health (mental and physical) takes precedence above everything else. Thus, if one's health is suffering, and one cannot eat and rest properly, it does not make sense to keep adding on activities, drive, etc.   First things first.

Use your parent logic. Make sure your messages and actions convey the degree to which you value your child's health above all else: more than grades, more than athletic performance, more than scholarships, etc.

Health is not negotiable, no matter how old your child is.

You wouldn't bargain with your child about the amount of illegal drugs they purchased, would you? You wouldn't discuss how much money they could steal from the local store? You wouldn't negotiate your child's mental or physical health? As such, your confident stance over what you child needs to do (i.e. a firm position), does not waiver, no matter how old your child is.

Are there differences when my child is older? What DOES differ is the amount of input they have in determining the path to health. Consider a clear, undisturbed, and firm approach with a young child, an adolescent, and an older (adult) child.

Child or Younger Adolescent --->

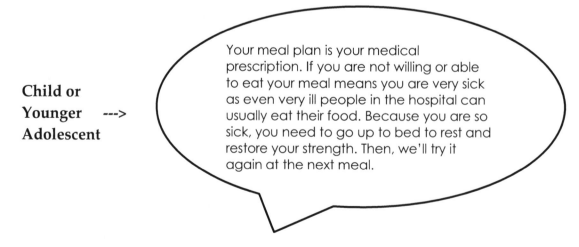

You realize, of course, since you are now a good behaviorist, you need to follow up

with the bedrest plan.

**Middle or
Older   --->
Adolescent**

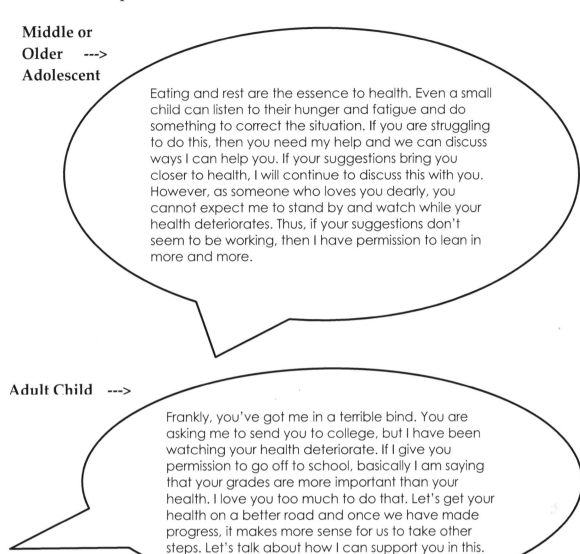

Eating and rest are the essence to health. Even a small child can listen to their hunger and fatigue and do something to correct the situation. If you are struggling to do this, then you need my help and we can discuss ways I can help you. If your suggestions bring you closer to health, I will continue to discuss this with you. However, as someone who loves you dearly, you cannot expect me to stand by and watch while your health deteriorates. Thus, if your suggestions don't seem to be working, then I have permission to lean in more and more.

Adult Child   --->

Frankly, you've got me in a terrible bind. You are asking me to send you to college, but I have been watching your health deteriorate. If I give you permission to go off to school, basically I am saying that your grades are more important than your health. I love you too much to do that. Let's get your health on a better road and once we have made progress, it makes more sense for us to take other steps. Let's talk about how I can support you in this.

Very Adult Child (i.e. child out of the house, on her or his own, etc.)

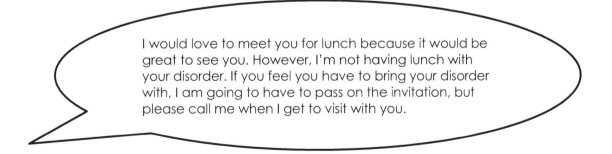

I would love to meet you for lunch because it would be great to see you. However, I'm not having lunch with your disorder. If you feel you have to bring your disorder with, I am going to have to pass on the invitation, but please call me when I get to visit with you.

Why do I consider these statements "firm?" They are said confidently, not in anger; not anxiously, just matter-of-fact and decisive. That is firmness.

F is for Funny. Funny? Why funny? How is this funny? Well, eating disorders certainly aren't funny, but this does not mean that humor does not have its place. Life is filled with pain. Pain makes life meaningful, strengthens our character, and teaches us valuable lessons about ourselves. However, to survive and live a meaningful life, we need to step back and find joy and laughter in everyday life. Humor and laughter is needed for many reasons.

~ We all need to be able to not take ourselves so seriously.

  o We need to roll with mistakes, laugh at some of the stupid things we all do, be able to take feedback, roll with the punches, and frankly, to laugh at all the ridiculous situations we get ourselves into as parents.

~ We need to be able to step back and laugh at some of the silly things this illness makes us do.

  o Did you ever dream you would be negotiating about rice cakes? Getting excited when your teenager ate a piece of chocolate? Monitoring bathroom use of an adult? This disorder puts families in some very odd situations.

~ We are going to keep making mistakes for as long as we live. We may as well accept that now.

  o Learning and growth are what make life interesting (in my opinion). How sad it would be to think we've "learned all there is to know." As a psychologist, I know I will always try to learn ways to be a more effective therapist and I would be irresponsible if I didn't. Silly to feel ashamed at what we don't know. Embrace our lapses, laugh, and learn, I say!!

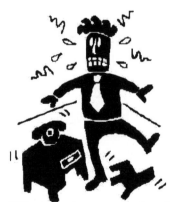

Off the C.U.F.F in Action: A Review

The Cleavers have a fourteen-year old daughter with anorexia nervosa. Because of the severity of her illness, their daughter, Eileen, has lost choice at mealtimes. It is dinnertime at the Cleaver household and Mrs. Cleaver is in the kitchen preparing dinner.

ENTER EILEEN.

Eileen: Are you using better to sauté those vegetables? If you put any butter on anything, I will not eat it.

Mrs. Cleaver does not look up from chopping vegetables and leans over and turns on the radio and starts humming along with the radio.

Eileen: Did you hear me?   I said I won't eat anything if you use butter.

Mrs. Cleaver chops away happily as it gets to the chorus.

Eileen: Forget it.   I'm not eating anything.

Eileen storms out of the kitchen.   Mrs. Cleaver, the quintessential housewife, proceeds to set the table. Fifteen minutes later, dinner is ready and Mrs. Cleaver summons the family. Eileen joins the rest of the family at dinner and proceeds to eat.

HUH?   I though she threatened she wasn't going to eat?

Explanation: We discuss this thoroughly in the chapter on behavior modification.   For now, think tantrum. A tantrum is a state of high emotional arousal. Think of yourself when you are in a high state of arousal (EXTREMELY ANGRY, EXTREMELY UPSET, etc.)   We call this "being on top of the emotional wave." Are you logical? Can you think clearly? Do you say extreme things to vent? Of course you do. Everybody does.

When your child's eating disorder is loud, s/he is in a high state of emotional arousal. Just like when we are upset, expressing our feelings, or "venting", can help to release these feelings. With an eating disorder, venting can take the form of threats, pre-meal obsessing about calories, hanging on the chef's shoulder and nagging, bargaining for smaller portions; the list goes on and on. As long as the parent remains calm and doesn't give in, such venting often passes and your child will resume eating with minimal further mishap.

Why did the parent do what she did?
Don't forget the golden rules. Mom was trying to not reinforce her child's eating disorder by giving it either positive attention (giving in to her daughter's request) or negative attention (yelling at her daughter for being a pain). Instead, she remained calm and in turn, her calmness helped Eileen to realize that there is nothing to be nervous about. Eileen was able to leave the situation and go calm down as well. **By remaining calm and unaffected, Mrs. Cleaver is communicating that there is nothing to be nervous about -a fact that is reassuring to her child.**

Putting New Management Strategies in Action: A Family Discussion

So, how do we go from where you are now with eating disorder management to get the family to work together as a team to fight this creature that has taken over your child? We have a family discussion, of course!

The purpose of a "family discussion" is to clearly communicate a "fresh start." Here are some questions I usually get around the notion of this family meeting, so I am giving you the question and answer section a little early this section.

Questions and Answers: The Family Discussion.

Q: When should I have a family discussion?

A: Probably a better question to ask is when shouldn't you have a family discussion? Communication is always essential. Talks are good. However, a good family talk about your child's disorder is particularly needed in the following:

→ Whenever you notice that it seems the family has gotten into a power struggle over disorder management (you have lost the family vs. the disorder formula and instead feel like it is your child against you).

→ You have been working at disorder management for a while and feel like everybody is stuck.

→ You find yourself getting burned out: like you are doing a lot of the work and don't feel that the other family members are doing their part. However, there is always a need to pause, take a step back and see how things are going, and make any changes necessary. The more you do this (talking about teamwork), the easier it gets. Trust your gut. When your worry meter is up, it's probably time for a talk.

Q: How should I do it? Should this be some "formal" discussion?

A: There really is no one answer for this one. How you do it is up to you, you know your family best. Here is what I have seen some families do:

→ Make an appointment with their child to talk.

→ Nail him or her when they have their child's attention during a long car ride.

→ Make checking-in part of a nightly routine.

→ Do it as part of an afternoon outing.

Q: Why am I doing this?

A: The overall purpose of this talk is to get your family united in helping your child to battle her/his disorder. The enlightening thing about managing an eating disorder is it serves as such a great demonstration of parenting. In parenting, you try something, you tweak your approach, you try again. The same thing goes for eating disorder management. You can't manage your child's eating disorder incorrectly. You will try a strategy as a family, you will give it a good try (not giving up because things get worse before they get better – they always do), you see what happens. If, over time, things are progressing, you keep going. If the approach could use a little tweaking, you tweak and go at it again.

Tips for Family Discussion

Over the years, I have collected strategies parents have found to be very helpful in managing their child's disorder. I summarize these in **Seven Rules**. First, I list the rules (some of them we've discussed already) and then I provide an explanation of the ones we haven't.

Mobilizing the Family as a Team to Fight the Disorder

Tips and Strategies

Rule #1 Externalize your child's disorder (explanation below).

Rule #2 Use your Off the C.U.F.F. approach.

Rule #3 Avoid a power struggle – it is the family against "it", the disorder, – not parents vs. child. If you find yourselves in a power struggle, it's time for a "time out" and another family meeting.

Rule #4 Be logical. Think developmental age, not chronological age.

Rule #5 Don't forget to reinforce the healthy coping behavior. Remember, eating disorders are coping strategies. We have to encourage and role model positive coping while we reduce unhealthy symptoms.

Rule #6 Take ownership of your own behavior and mistakes. Change starts with you. The more willing you are to admit mistakes, and to make personal changes to lead a more balanced and healthy lifestyle, the more willing your child is going to be.

Rule #7 Parents have more options than they think. Unless your child is financially independent, you have the ability to communicate health as the priority before grades, before activities – just communicate these things using support and concern - not through threats and bullying.

Rule #1 Externalize Your Child's Disorder

Why?

Externalizing the disorder helps you to understand what your child is going through, helps you to not blame your child, and helps to avoid conflict because you and your child are joined together to fight this common enemy. By externalizing the disorder, we mean that you should consider the eating disorder as something separate from your child. Indeed, this is what your child experiences. When you externalize the disorder, you help to create a concrete thing that the whole family can bond together and fight!

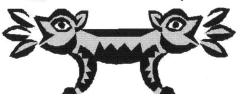

How?

Visualize the disorder. Here is an example:

Visualizing the disorder as a separate monster can help you from being critical of your child while helping you target your negative energy to the source that deserves it – the eating disorder. If it is helpful, visualize the eating disorder to be someone who you or your child can't stand!! I usually picture the

disorder as a big pimple. Yes, I know, I'm a professional.

Name the disorder. Some people find it helpful to give the disorder a name. This can help you to remember that the disorder is not your child. It is a THING that your child is struggling with. Some people prefer just to refer to it as "the eating disorder."

As you can imagine, this is a developmentally sensitive strategy. The young children I work with like it, the adolescents think it is "so dumb" and the adults really get into it. However, this shouldn't stop you from referring to "the disorder" or "your burden" or "your guilt machine" – or whatever. Ask your child; he or she will tell you what they like.

Your name is Joe, Joe the disorder; otherwise known as "the dark side."

Here are some examples of what this strategy would look like if you implemented it at home.

Examples of referring to your child's disorder as separate.

Scene 1   The Dinner Table.

Child: No, I won't eat that and you can't make me.

Parent: I am not negotiating with an eating disorder. Let's both calm down and we'll go at it again together.

Scene 2   The Dinner Table (the next night).

Child: I hate you. If you loved me, you wouldn't make me eat this.

Parent: I love you. I hate the eating disorder. Because I love you, the eating disorder isn't getting an inch. Let's eat.

Scene 3   Your child is getting dressed for the day.

Child: I am so fat! Everyone will hate me.

Parent: Your eating disorder is shouting at you again. We need to leave here in 10 minutes. Then we can figure out what is really going on as we're driving to school.

Basically your attitude is to listen attentively to your child, but not the disorder. Anything the disorder has to say not only is of no interest to you, but it bores you and is not worth your time. I like to imagine the voice of the eating disorder as an annoying gnat that keeps flying at your ear that you mindlessly swat away without further attention. However, often your best strategy is just ignoring the disorder altogether. For this strategy to work best, you need to warn your child this is what you WILL be doing

the next time the disorder is loud – ignoring it because it only hurts your child. It is not fair to introduce this strategy "all of a sudden." After you have ignored it in the moment, later, when the intensity has passed, go and talk to your child and explore upsetting things that may have happened during the day that made him/her upset. Eating disorders are coping strategies. They get louder when other things are going on.

✿ Perfectionist's Corner ✿

<u>Perfectionist</u>:   My child gets very upset before mealtimes (or after mealtimes – or both). How am I being a good parent if I am causing her to do things that upset her?

<u>Voice of Reason</u>: A good parent not only strives to create a sense of safety for her child. He/she also must teach her child how to manage when life gets difficult.   Individuals feel much more able to cope with the world when they feel they have the skills to cope no matter what happens.   People often experience a great deal of distress when they expect the world to operate in a certain way and it doesn't conform to their expectations.

SOLUTION: By learning to cope with stress of her eating disorder, your child will learn how to cope with stress in general.   These skills will go a long way in helping her to be successful in whatever she chooses to pursue.

Friendly reminder: This is not a power struggle.

Remember, you and your child are united in fighting a common enemy: the eating disorder. At times when the eating disorder is loud, it may FEEL like a power struggle. At those times, use the strategies we talked about (also see emotional wave pages), offer encouragement, and seek support.

Oftentimes parents get confused because their child has difficulty determining where they end and the eating disorder begins – they think they ARE their eating disorder. Thus, when they are listening to their eating disorder, they feel they are FINALLY doing something for themselves. This is a particularly important issue for someone with an eating disorder as often they have never done things for themselves – they are too busy pleasing everybody else.

However, when they think that listening to their eating disorder is listening to their "true inner self" they are mistaken. Their true inner self, the kind and caring parent that we have spoken of, would not be trying to harm them, would it?

Thus, when adolescents say they feel that listening to the eating disorder is the only thing they have "control" over, I usually explain the following. I explain that an eating disorder is like having an evil tyrant in their heads. It doesn't take guts or courage to go along with

the crowd and follow the dictator. Rather, true courage is fighting back and speaking out. Following the voice of a dictator, their eating disorder, is not TRUE control. Control is the ability to be flexible in challenging situations, to roll with the punches, to problem solve, and to have the courage to try new things. For whatever reason, your child has not yet mastered these skills and, instead, uses their disorder as a coping strategy. Fighting back against their disorder is a way for them to take control for once in their life!!

E.D. is not allowing Lauren control but fighting back will

Key Points

I warned you…this was a doozy of a section! Here are all the things we learned.

  i. An Off the C.U.F.F. approach is a great style to practice in managing your child's eating disorder.
  ii. This is a family mission: the whole family bonding together to battle this disorder.
  iii. Discuss strategies and seek your child's input AS LONG AS that input comes from a place of health and not illness. There is no negotiation with an eating disorder, but your child can give healthy input.
  iv. Consider your child's age in the degree of input, but don't miscommunicate your values. Health comes first.
  v. Whenever the plan is unclear, it's time to regroup and replan (otherwise known as a "family discussion, a family car ride, a letter to your child – do what works).
  vi. Your child is not his or her disorder – no matter what s/he feels in the moment. When the eating disorder is loud, that is a moment of extreme emotional intensity for your child and they may not have clarity.

Weekly Goals

We start our full homework this week! Using what you have learned about your child's symptoms and the skills s/he needs to develop, we'll make some weekly goals. Tips for completing the homework sheet and two blank sheets (one for you, one for your support person), are found on the following pages.

Homework Tips

1) Be specific and describe BEHAVIORS your child does. This makes it much easier to think of a plan.

2) For each step, write both WHAT BEHAVIOR you will target and HOW you will do it.

3) Think through BARRIERS that might get in the way of accomplishing your goals. If you think through the things that might get in the way, it will help you to deal with these things when they happen.

4) I am serious about doing something nice for yourself. VERY SERIOUS.

5) We target unhealthy behaviors in levels. We start with the behaviors that are most harmful to health. Only after we are out of danger do we shift our focus in Step One.

Wisdom of the Week: My Gift to Myself

Look in the mirror and smile. You used to do it when you were a child. You deserve it just as much now.   Oh yeah, go back to the chair.

GOALS FOR WEEK #2

Date:

Remember our key guidelines
It's a process! Try, tweak, grow and learn.
Self-parenting: a necessary prerequisite for other parenting.
Learn how to SURF The WAVE!
Remain genuine.

Unhealthy or unhelpful behavior I will discuss WITH my child this week and our plan to address it.

Eats too little	✗Eats too little variety	Exercises too much
Throws up after meals	Doesn't get enough sleep	Doesn't set limits
Abuses laxatives	Engages in self-harm	Other

Possible Suggestions of How to Address:	My Plan:
☐ Ignore it ☐ Have a discussion about needed change in behavior *(discuss a future, necessary, logical consequence given the severity of the behavior)* ☐ Implement a logical consequence (reminding your child of the importance of health before anything) ☐ Appeal to your child's inner wisdom (have a discussion with your child about what you have observed, why you are concerned, the change in behavior expected) ☐ Reverse Time-Out (you leave) ☐ Group Time-Out (everyone leaves for 10 minutes) ☐ Regrouping (family meeting to get out of power struggle) ☐ Humor	Would a discussion be a good idea?

Heathy Coping Strategy I will address with my child this week and my plan to address it.

Express negative emotions effectively	Ask for more help	Set more limits (cut down study time, set a regular bedtime, cut out an activity)
Express an opinion- even if someone may disagree	Be more considerate of others	Place more realistic demands on oneself (consider the cost, not whether the demands are achieved)
Get a better balance of work and leisure	View a situation with curiosity rather than with criticism	Manage disappointing results
Share a vulnerability with someone	Embrace and learn from mistakes rather than running from them	Resolve a conflict
Tune in and respond more to what your feelings are telling you	Take more pride in oneself (being a more respectful self-parent)	Strut
Be Silly or just take yourself less seriously	Smile at your reflection	Initiate plans
Try something new	Get Messy	Break a ritual
Get more sleep	Other	Other

Possible Suggestions:	My Plan:
☐ Positive attention when takes a step toward behavior ☐ One-on-one time outside of eating disorder stuff ☐ Earning a logical privilege given increased health ☐ Praise and STOP – no BUTS ☐ Role Model Behavior Yourself ☐ Open the door for a discussion ☐ Set a limit ☐ Offer to teach ☐ Other	

Heathy Coping Strategy I will Role Model this week.

Possible Suggestions:	My Plan:
☐ Delegate something. ☐ Say 'no' to some things. ☐ Be honest with my feelings. ☐ Express my feelings when not on the wave. ☐ Ask for help. ☐ Set healthy limits between my needs and those of others. ☐ Listen with full attention. ☐ Praise and STOP. ☐ Say "I'm sorry" with no excuses. ☐ Allow family members to make mistakes without jumping in. ☐ Be consistent. ☐ Address negative self-talk. ☐ Be reliable.	

Self-care Strategy I will implement this week

Possible Suggestions:	My Plan:
☐ Make regular mealtimes a priority. ☐ Set a regular bedtime. ☐ Learn a new hobby. ☐ Spend some time with my friends. ☐ Spend time ALONE with my spouse. ☐ Set a regular time I stop work each day. ☐ Take weekends off. ☐ Buy something for myself. ☐ Exercise in a MODERATE manner. ☐ Take pride in my physical appearance.	No lame excuses!!

TIP OF THE WEEK: Exit if you need to, but do it in style.

CHAPTER THREE: Tricks to Implementing Your Approach

Where You Are

- ✓ You have finished your first step.   You have learned more about the program.

- ✓ You have learned more about the stages of parenting and how eating disorders take your child off the path of healthy growth.

- ✓ You have learned a general approach to eating disorder management.

- ✓ You have learned how eating disorders serve as coping strategies.

- ✓ You have begun to get an idea of the targets you need to work on and have mobilized your family to start tackling these goals one at a time.

- ✓ You are beginning to appreciate the importance of yourself as a role model.

Congratulations.

Topic: Tricks and Strategies (Learning to Surf the Emotional Wave)

We have given you a lot of information about the nature of your child's disorder. We described the steps we need to go through to help the family get healthier, and we discussed an approach that can be effective with implementation: Off the C.U.F.F. It is the "U" part of C.U.F.F., being **undisturbed**, that we discuss in this chapter. These disorders are so upsetting and/or frustrating sometimes (all the time?) that remaining undisturbed is difficult. I want to give you five good reasons why remaining undisturbed is important (some of this is review, but it's important).

1. Learning to remain calm in the face of stress helps you manage stress better.

2. Learning to remain calm requires you to effectively control, understand, and express your feelings. By learning to do this, you become a master "emotion regulator."

3. Regulating and understanding emotions builds self-trust, self-confidence, and self-knowledge.

4. Once you learn this, you can role model for your children and teach it to your children (not to say you are not doing this already!).

5. Your children are NOT good "emotion regulators." This is one skill deficit that keeps the eating
disorder
going.

The Emotional Wave

HOW? Well, let me introduce you to the "Emotional Wave."

An Intimate Moment with the Emotional Wave.

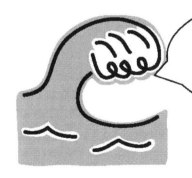

Why, hello. I am the Emotional Wave. I like to wreak havoc on your daily existence.

Emotions are like waves. Waves are a useful comparison because waves rise and fall and come and go just as moods do. Some people are more "emotional" than others (their waves go higher or they may rise and fall more quickly). Just as it is easier to navigate through a calm sea rather than a tidal wave, so emotions of medium strength are easier to manage than REALLY INTENSE emotions. However, just as a completely calm sea is rather boring, so do emotions add excitement and color to life!

Regardless of whether you sail on a relatively calm sea or whether you find yourself living in more volatile waters, the goals are the same. The more you learn about waves, the better you can navigate – no matter what the journey is like! Using this logic, we will teach you how to use your feelings to help you and your child get through this illness and to improve life in general!

TIP BOX

Emotions can be wonderful when we learn to listen to, and understand, the information they provide to us. When you don't understand emotions – their purpose, what they tell us, how to use that information – emotions can seem complicated and overwhelming.

We don't go into great detail about emotions here. We save that for later. The focus of this section is to give you some quick fixes. These fixes are intended to help you control your own emotions so that extremely strong emotions do not get in the way of your ability to help your child. Later on, we focus on developing emotion regulation skills in your child.

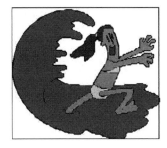

Your Mission:

◊   Get yourself off the top of the wave with minimal injury.
◊   Be alert to tidal waves.
◊   Feel confident in surfing waves.
◊   Teach your child how to surf.

Why Should I Bother Learning to Surf?

Let's consider a before and after scenario.

BEFORE: MEET MR. "I'M NEVER ANGRY." Mr. I'm Never Angry has trouble speaking out for what he wants because he feels that if people really cared about him, they would know what he needed. As a result he is continually disappointed. Rather than express his disappointment, he lets the anger build up over time. Periodically, he reaches a breaking point when all that pent up anger comes crashing out – his TIDAL WAVE. The problem is that the trigger for the tidal wave is usually something minor. This makes Mr. I'm Never Angry look ridiculous as his justified feelings of anger come out in a relatively minor situation.

HERE'S WHAT WE MEAN: THE TIDAL WAVE.
Mr. I'm Never Angry loves to go with his family to the beach. His wife is a real estate agent. Her income supplements the family and is budgeted for "extras" – family vacations, etc. For three weekends, Mr. I'm Never Angry has mentioned that the family

has not been to the beach in a while, but Mrs. I'm Never Angry keeps scheduling house showings on the weekends. Mr. I'm Never Angry gets more and more hurt and angry believing that if his wife really cared about him, she would schedule her showings for another time. Finally, the tidal wave crashes when Mrs. I'm Just Trying to Please My Husband is 15 minutes late one night due to her job.

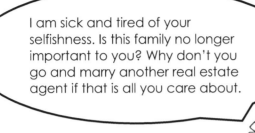

> I am sick and tired of your selfishness. Is this family no longer important to you? Why don't you go and marry another real estate agent if that is all you care about.

> Huh?? I am 15 minutes late. What is your problem?

THE EXPLOSION

So what are the problems?

→ Mr. I'm Never Angry could use some help in making specific requests like, "Honey, let's go to the beach this weekend. Can you rearrange your schedule so we can go?"

→ Mr. I'm Never Angry could use some help recognizing signs of irritation so he can address his anger when it is starting to increase rather than waiting for the tidal wave.

→ Because he finally exploded over a relatively minor matter, Mr. I'm Never Angry looks silly when, actually, his original complaint was legitimate.

→ Mrs. I'm Never Angry could work on being more validating of her husband's anger rather than critical.

AFTER PHOTO: IT COULD HAVE BEEN LIKE THIS. So what's another way this scenario could have turn out if Mr. I'm Never Angry worked on his emotion regulation skills?

→ He would have recognized he was getting irritated and tried to figure out why.

→ He would have realized that his wife's weekend schedule was making him feel neglected.

→ He would have spoken out.

→ His wife, who was working because she thought her husband really liked her too, would have realized her misinterpretation and would have changed her work schedule.

...and everyone would live happily ever after.

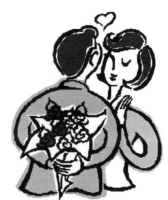

This is what we are aiming for. Let's show you how.

Step One: Notice the signs that you are starting to climb the wave and act immediately.

The first step in mastering waves is learning to notice signs that the waves are starting to get higher. I often have individuals report they go from no anger to extreme anger instantly. However, once we start exploring this further, we learn that when you start to pay attention, there are subtle signs that your emotions are getting more intense.

Why is important to notice these subtle signs? Well, at the lower levels of the wave you can still think clearly. It is more likely that you will be effective. At the top of the wave, logic is gone and it is more likely that you will do and say something stupid, or worse, something destructive.

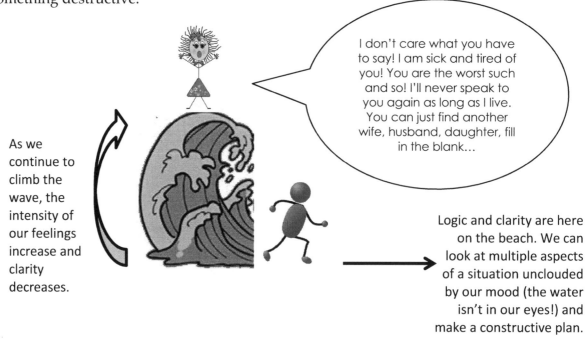

As we continue to climb the wave, the intensity of our feelings increase and clarity decreases.

I don't care what you have to say! I am sick and tired of you! You are the worst such and so! I'll never speak to you again as long as I live. You can just find another wife, husband, daughter, fill in the blank...

Logic and clarity are here on the beach. We can look at multiple aspects of a situation unclouded by our mood (the water isn't in our eyes!) and make a constructive plan.

Learning the Signs: Introduction to Emotions

So how does one notice the wave starting to grow? Well, you start by being an observer of your own behavior. To understand what you should be looking FOR, you need a little information about emotions.

Emotions are made up of three primary components:
1) We have certain sensations in our body.
2) We think certain types of thoughts.
3) We have the URGE to do certain things.

TIP BOX

Researchers believe all these changes occur in our body, mind, and action urges because emotions communicate a need. If we pay attention to our feelings, learn the need being communicated, and take effective steps to meet that need, the emotion will end. We will learn later the different function of different emotions.

Let's think of an example:

SADNESS

1. BODY SENSATION – You may feel weary and tired. Your arms and legs may feel heavy and you may feel like you have to drag your body form place to place.

2. THOUGHTS – You may have negative thoughts about yourself, think about all the mistakes you have made since the first day you were born, and predict that all the most negative things will happen in the future.

3. ACTION URGE – You may have the urge to be by yourself and not do anything. Action urges are important because they help us figure out the need our emotion is communicating. However, when we act on the urge at the top of wave, we don't get our needs met effectively. We get our needs met destructively. That's the problem. We need to listen to the messages of our feelings when we have clarity so we act on the messages of our emotions without causing harm… to ourselves or people we care about. In the case of sadness, the need is comfort. We need to be soothing ourselves either by stepping back from responsibilities and nurturing ourselves or by reaching out to others.

TIP BOX

If we start noticing the other two parts: the sensations in our bodies and characteristic thoughts, then we can stop the wave in its tracks.

Everybody is different. You may notice the feelings in your body first or there may be certain thoughts that serve as your trigger. What follows is a list of strategies to try, depending on the things you notice first: your body or your thoughts.

Step Two: Use a strategy to bring yourself down from the top of the wave or to keep yourself from going there in the first place.

STRATEGY #1:   SELF-SOOTHING

When should you use this strategy?
When the first thing you notice is THE WAY YOUR BODY FEELS.
POINT: IF YOU CAN MAKE YOUR BODY FEEL DIFFERENTY, YOU CAN HELP TO CHANGE YOUR MOOD! In addition, self-soothing can be a powerful way to bring yourself down from the top of the wave!

You are trying to improve the way your body feels in the moment. Think of the sense of touch. You are trying to FEEL better in the physical sense so engaging in an activity that appeals to the sense of touch is appropriate here.

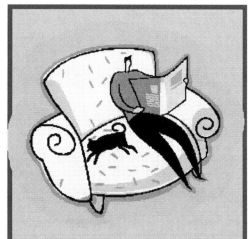

- o   Take a bubble bath
- o   Have a massage
- o   Put creamy lotion on your whole body

Off the C.U.F.F. Tricks to Implement Your Approach
- o   Put a cold compress on your forehead
- o   Sink into a really comfortable chair at home
- o   Put on a silky blouse or pair of pajamas
- o   Wrap yourself in a flannel robe
- o   Take a hot, hot shower
- o   Put a pair of tennis balls on the floor and roll your back on them to get those knots out of your back.
- o   Roll your feet on some golf balls (trust me on this one)
- o   Brush your hair for a long time (or get your child to brush your hair)
- o   Get someone to tickle your back
- o   Blow dry your feet
- o   TAKE SLOW, DEEP, BREATHS FROM YOUR DIAPHRAGMS or try one of the breathing exercises on the next page.

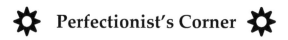 **Perfectionist's Corner**

Perfectionist: I tried one of the strategies.   It didn't work. I've always been this way. It's hopeless to change.

Voice of Reason: Managing emotions takes practice, lots of practice. Don't give up on a strategy if you've just tried it once. You may have to try it several times. In addition, certain strategies work at certain times, so you may have to have a variety of strategies in your toolbox.

Breathing and Stretching Activities to Relax Your Body

When your body lives in a constant state of tension, you often don't realize how tight your muscles have become. If this is the case for you, you may not notice subtle increases in muscle tension that alert you to a worsening in mood. To help with this, a strategy called "progressive muscle relaxation" was developed. This strategy asks people to work through each muscle group by stressing and relaxing each muscle group. I like to follow script because the imagery really helps to contract those muscles. It was developed for children, so it would also be a great script to use with your children. Some people find it helpful to tape record the script so that they can play the tape and practice the imagery.

The Script: Progressive Muscle Relaxation for Children
Author Unknown

Introduction

Today we're going to practice some special kinds of exercises called relaxation exercises. These exercises help you to learn how to relax when you're feeling uptight and help you get rid of those butterflies-in-your-stomach kinds of feelings. They're also kind of neat because you can learn how to do some of them without anyone really noticing. In order for you to get the best feelings from these exercises, there are some rules you must follow. First, you must do exactly what I say, even if it seems kind of silly. Second, you must try hard to do what I say. Third, you must pay attention to your body. Throughout these exercises, pay attention to how your muscles feel when they are tight and when they are loose and relaxed. And fourth, you must practice. The more you practice, the more relaxed you can get. Do you have any questions? Are you ready to begin? Okay, first, get as comfortable as you can in your chair. Sit back, get both feet on the floor, and just let your arms hang loose. That's fine. Now close your eyes and don't open them until I say to. Remember to follow my instructions very carefully, try hard, and pay attention to your body. Here we go.

Hands and Arms

Pretend you have a whole lemon in your left hand. Now squeeze it hard. Try to squeeze all the juice out. Feel the tightness in your hand and arm as you squeeze. Now drop the lemon. Notice how your muscles feel when they are relaxed. Take another lemon and squeeze. Try to squeeze this one harder than you did the first one. That's right. Real hard. Now drop the lemon and relax. See how much better your hand and arm feel when they are relaxed. Once again, take a lemon in your left hand and squeeze all the juice out. Don't leave a single drop. Squeeze hard. Good. Now relax and let the lemon fall from your hand. (Repeat the process for the right hand and arm.)

Arms and Shoulders

Pretend you are a furry, lazy cat. You want to stretch. Stretch your arms out in front of you. Raise them up high over your head. Way back. Feel the pull in your shoulders. Stretch higher. Now just let your arms drop back to your side. Okay, kitten, let's stretch again. Stretch your arms out in front of you. Raise them over your head. Pull them back, way back. Pull hard. Now let them drop quickly. Good. Notice how your shoulders feel more relaxed. This time let's have a great big stretch. Try to touch the ceiling. Stretch your arms way out in front of you. Raise them way up high over your head. Push them way, way back. Notice the tension and pull in your arms and shoulders. Hold tight, now. Great. Let them drop very quickly and feel how good it is to be relaxed. It feels good and warm and lazy.

Jaw

You have a giant jawbreaker bubble gum in your mouth. It's very hard to chew. Bite down on it. Hard! Let your neck muscles help you. Now relax. Just let your jaw hang loose. Notice that how good it feels just to let your jaw drop. Okay, let's tackle that jawbreaker again now. Bite down. Hard! Try to squeeze it out between your teeth. That's good. You're really tearing that gum up. Now relax again. Just let your jaw drop off your face. It feels good just to let go and not have to fight that bubble gum. Okay, one more time. We're really going to tear it up this time. Bite down. Hard as you can. Harder. Oh, you're really working hard. Good. Now relax. Try to relax your whole body. You've beaten that bubble gum. Let yourself go as loose as you can.

Stomach

Hey! Here comes a cute baby elephant. But he's not watching where he's going. He doesn't see you lying in the grass, and he's about to step on your stomach. Don't move. You don't have time to get out of the way. Just get ready for him. Make your stomach very hard. Tighten up your stomach muscles real tight. Hold it. It looks like he is going the other way. You can relax now. Let your stomach go soft. Let it be as relaxed as you can. That feels so much better. Oops, he's coming this way again. Get Ready. Tighten up your stomach. Real hard. If he steps on you when your stomach is hard, it won't hurt. Make your stomach into a rock. Okay, he's moving away again. You can relax now. Kind of settle down, get comfortable, and relax. Notice the difference between a tight stomach and a relaxed one. That's how we want to feel—nice and loose and relaxed. You won't believe this, but this time he's coming your way and no turning around. He's headed straight for you. Tighten up. Tighten hard. Here he comes. This is really it. You've got to hold on tight. He's stepping on you. He's stepped over you. Now he's gone for good. You can relax completely. You're safe. Everything is okay, and you can feel nice and relaxed.

Legs and Feet

Now pretend that you are standing barefoot in a big, fat mud puddle. Squish your toes down deep into the mud. Try to get your feet down to the bottom of the mud puddle. You'll probably need your legs to help you push. Push down, spread your toes apart, feel the mud squish up between your toes. Now step out of the mud puddle. Relax your feet. Let your toes go loose and feel how nice that it feels to be relaxed. Back into the mud puddle. Squish your toes down. Let your leg muscles help push your feet down. Push your feet. Hard. Try to squeeze that puddle dry. Okay. Come back out now. Relax your feet, relax your legs, relax your toes. It feels so good to be relaxed. No tenseness anywhere. You feel kind of warm and tingly.

Conclusion

Stay as relaxed as you can. Let your whole body go limp and feel all your muscles relaxed. In a few minutes I will ask you to open your eyes, and that will be the end of this practice session. As you go through the day, remember how good it feels to be relaxed. Sometimes you have to make yourself tighter before you can be relaxed, just as we did in these exercises. Practice these exercises every day to get more and more relaxed. A good time to practice is at night, after you have gone to bed and the lights are out and you won't be disturbed. It will help you get to sleep. Then, when you are really a good relaxer, you can help yourself relax at school. Just remember the elephant, or the jaw breaker, or the mud puddle, and you can do our exercises and nobody will know. Today is a good day, and you are ready to feel very relaxed. You've worked hard and it feels good to work hard. Very slowly, now, open your eyes and wiggle your muscles around a little. Very good. You've done a good job. You're going to be a super relaxer.

STRATEGY #2:   DISTRACTION

When Should You Use This Strategy?

When the first thing you usually notice is YOUR THOUGHTS GETTING MORE AND MORE EMOTIONAL.

TIP BOX

If you can focus your mental energy on something else for a little while, it will help you calm down. You will then be able to view the situation with greater clarity and can use your problem solving skills.

Distraction Strategies

Go for a drive.	Play pool.
Pretend you are buying a new car and go for a test drive.	Throw a tennis ball against the garage door.
Browse around a bookstore.	Do a crossword puzzle.
Dust.	Play computer games.
Make some homemade bread.	Dress up and look nice.
Plan a picnic.	Buy something for yourself (jewelry, shoes)
Go to the park.	Talk on the phone.
Spend a few hours in a library with a good book.	Pick a foreign language you would like to learn and find a class or tape.
Walk around an art museum.	Talk on the phone.
Say "I love you".	Think about your good qualities.
Go bowling.	Go on a bike ride.
Fantasize about life getting better.	Get your hair cut.
Take a sports, dance or music lesson.	Make a list of things you want to do.
Care for your pets.	Make a photo album.
Exercise.	Do a word puzzle.
Talk with a friend or relative.	Soak in the bathtub.
Sing.	Go to a movie.
Go to the beach.	Take a walk.
Go rollerblading or roller skating.	Listen to music.
Play a musical instrument.	Lie in the sun (don't forget your sunscreen)
Make a gift for someone.	Read a magazine.
Buy a CD.	Look at photos.
Put on some good blues music.	Make a scrapbook.
Walk around the mall.	Go shoot a basketball.
Draw or doodle.	Vacuum.
Write a short story.	Plan a party.
Plan a day trip.	Watch sports on television.
Plan a long trip.	Make a new CD of your favorite music.
Plan a year long trip & imagine yourself without children!	Reorganize a cabinet or closet that is driving you crazy.

Putting it all Together: Surfing the Emotional Wave

1. Notice the signs that you are starting to get upset or agitated (or, if too late, notice that you are on top of the wave).

2. Try a strategy to bring you down from the top of the wave. Note: Don't get discouraged as this takes practice. Over time, you will learn what works and when it works.

3. When you feel that you are level-headed, you in a position to begin to think of solutions to the dilemma that began to get you upset in the first place. Your emotions were trying to tell you something: now is the time to figure it out.

4. Consider your feelings, think through the dilemma, and approach the problem.

5. Try your strategy. See what happens. Learn from what happens.

6. Tweak your approach and try again.

7. Congratulate yourself on getting through a difficult situation with minimal damage.

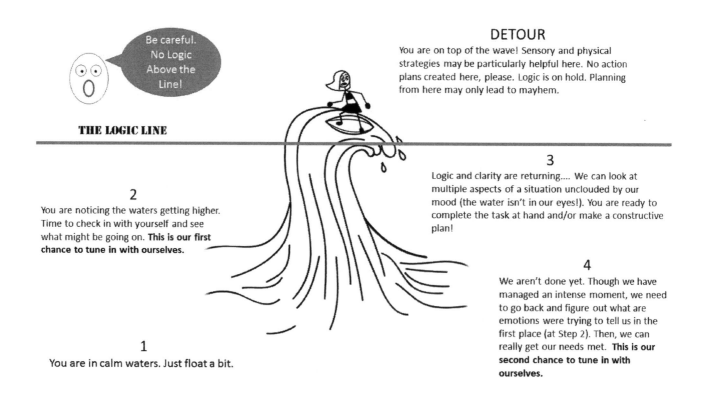

The Emotional Wave

Mastering the Emotional Wave: Step by Step

Let's take a look at what mastering the wave would look like in practice and how you would implement the various suggestions we have mentioned at each level of the wave.

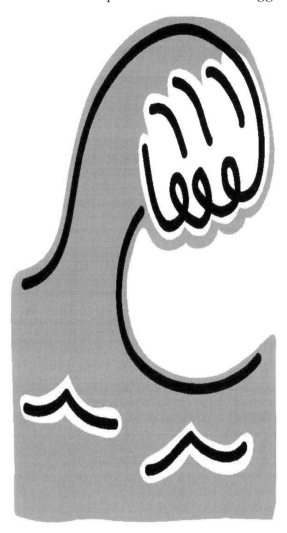

You are at the top of the wave

Your level of emotional energy is too strong to think clearly. You will need to lower the intensity BEFORE you do anything else. Strategies that demand a lot of concentration (playing games, reading, etc.) won't work well here.   It is often best to leave the situation WITH DIGNITY and then do some calming strategies (a walk, deep breathing, driving if OK to drive).

Your level of emotional energy is almost maxed out. It is difficult to think clearly here so you do not want to be thinking through solutions to your problems or giving others advice here.   You may have a hard time using strategies to calm yourself down that require concentration (e.g. reading, word puzzles). You may have better luck with things that ABRUPTLY snap you out of it (driving and playing really loud music – blues preferred, a comedian on TV, a really HOT shower).   When you have regained some clarity, time to think!
As your level of emotional energy goes up, use strategies that require less concentration.

Your level of emotional energy is definitely up, although you still have the ability to concentrate. A wide range of strategies could be used here: distraction, relaxation, etc.   Check in with yourself to see if you REALLY can look at the situation without your emotions biasing what you see. If you can be objective, go into problem-solving mode. If not, stick with a strategy a while longer. Emotion regulation sometimes takes a bit.

The lower your emotional intensity, the more options are available to you. Careful though. Don't go into "problem solving" until you REALLY have mental clarity.

You notice your level of emotional energy starting to rise. Good for you! You have complete clarity and can do some self-coaching to figure out why you might be upset. Separate those aspects of the situation you have control over versus the aspects you need to work to accept. Make a plan to address the aspects you can affect. Use your wave skills to help tolerate the negative feelings that arise from accepting the aspects you can't do anything about.

**Good problem solving involves separating the aspects of a situation you have control over from those you don't. You make a plan to address the aspects you can influence.
You work on accepting the aspects you don't.**

You are on the beach.   Just revel in it!

TIP BOX

A Few Words on Control and Acceptance

On the bottom step of the wave in the above diagram, I mention separating those aspects of a situation that you have control over, and accepting those aspects that you don't. To be able to do this, first you have to have a clear idea of what you have control over. Frankly, not much. You control what you do, i.e. your behavior. You can't control your thoughts. You CAN control how you react to your thoughts. You can control how you treat others. Your behavior can INCREASE THE LIKELIHOOD that individuals respond in certain ways, but it does not guarantee they will.

When we can't control a situation that is very upsetting, this is incredibly difficult. We can't stop thinking about it and we often have trouble not worrying about it. Our first step in managing this situation is taking a step back, and looking at the situation with clear vision. Then, ask yourself the following question:

1. Have I done everything I can do in this situation? Think about: role modeling effective coping, expressing your emotions effectively, treating others consistently, following up on rules and contingencies…etc.

If so, then the ball is in the other person's court. It becomes a matter of tolerating distress and using your wave strategies: distraction or soothing. It also helps to repeat the following about 20 million times a minute:

"I wish I could do something more about this situation. I will continue to take control of what I can: my effectiveness, my self-care, and my consistency and trust in the process. If I keep this up, things are most likely to turn out. In the meantime, I will keep it up, gather support from loved ones, and keep my sanity."

The Emotional Wave for Your Child

Does the emotional wave make sense? I hope so because I am about to make things a little bit more complicated. Your child is not good at identifying his or her feelings. Instead of reading the feelings DIRECTLY, your child uses an INTERPRETER: THE EATING DISORDER.

For this to make sense, let's first think of a situation not related to eating disorders you may have experienced. Imagine you wake up one morning and you are in a sad and lonely mood. As a result, you don't start your day on the beach. Rather, you have already started climbing the wave (though certainly you still have some distance to the top). When we have started climbing, sometimes it seems as if we have a filter on what we see: we see the world through the lens of our mood. Our mood colors are what we focus on, what we pay attention to, and how we view things (you've heard of "rose-colored" glasses? Same principle). In other words, we tend to focus on things in our environment that STRENGTHEN or at least VALIDATE our mood.

For example, when we start off the day sad and lonely, our filter focuses on all the times in the day when we are alone and our filter tends to disregard or ignore those times when we are with others.

SO, on this particular morning, given your mood, you walk past an office worker who does not speak to you. Now, on any other morning when this has happened, you wouldn't think twice about it. You might think "She must be busy." BUT, because of your sad and lonely filter, you might think "Oh goodness. She's mad at me. I wonder why she is avoiding me. A lot of people seem to be avoiding me. I must not be very likeable."

You get the picture. A similar thing happens to your child. When your child begins to climb the wave because of something TRULY upsetting (THE REAL EVENT), s/he has the EATING DISORDER FILTER activated. As a result, your child becomes more sensitive to eating and weight issues that s/he would be able to tolerate on a day on the beach.

Take home point: negative moods sensitize your child to eating disorder related things in the environment and these eating disorder things finish the job and send your child to the top of the wave.

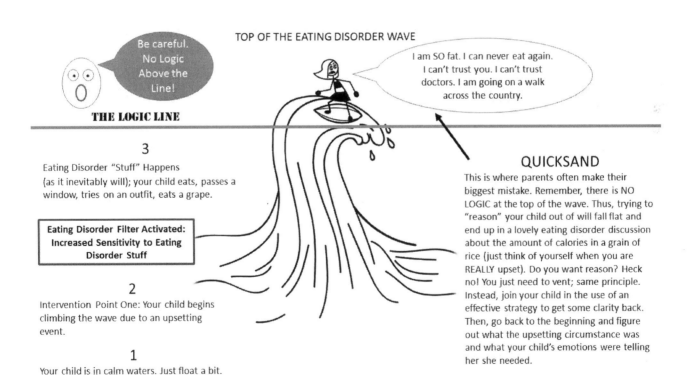

TOP OF THE EATING DISORDER WAVE

Be careful. No Logic Above the Line!

I am SO fat. I can never eat again. I can't trust you. I can't trust doctors. I am going on a walk across the country.

THE LOGIC LINE

3
Eating Disorder "Stuff" Happens (as it inevitably will); your child eats, passes a window, tries on an outfit, eats a grape.

Eating Disorder Filter Activated: Increased Sensitivity to Eating Disorder Stuff

2
Intervention Point One: Your child begins climbing the wave due to an upsetting event.

1
Your child is in calm waters. Just float a bit.

QUICKSAND
This is where parents often make their biggest mistake. Remember, there is NO LOGIC at the top of the wave. Thus, trying to "reason" your child out of will fall flat and end up in a lovely eating disorder discussion about the amount of calories in a grain of rice (just think of yourself when you are REALLY upset). Do you want reason? Heck no! You just need to vent; same principle. Instead, join your child in the use of an effective strategy to get some clarity back. Then, go back to the beginning and figure out what the upsetting circumstance was and what your child's emotions were telling her she needed.

Once the ED filter is activated by some upsetting event, an "eating disorder issue" may trigger a further rise in the wave, and EVENTUALLY, an "EATING DISORDER TIDAL WAVE." This is one of the ways the eating disorder serves as a coping strategy for your child. Negative emotional energy, caused for WHATEVER reason, is channeled through the filter of the EATING DISORDER and the "real problem" is replaced with an eating disorder issue. Why? For many reasons, but for one, worrying about weight and physical appearance is concrete and in your child's opinion, may be under "his or her control." In contrast, most upsetting events in life are NOT under our control, we just have to tolerate the distress caused by them if we can't "fix them." Thus, your child has taken an uncontrollable problem and turned it into a controllable problem. Pretty clever, huh?

The problem of course is that the REAL problem doesn't get addressed and your child's health gets impaired. HMMMM. Maybe NOT so clever. This is confusing for parents because when you ask your child what is wrong, s/he will say, "I ate too much, I feel fat, etc.." when a REAL incident that happened earlier MAY be the true source of woe. The eating disorder filter just gave them the ability to channel that negative emotional energy into eating related stuff. Confused? Walk through the diagram on the previous page and see if it makes sense for you.

This can give you a very POWERFUL treatment strategy if you understand that when your child seems to be in "eating disorder mode" it is because something is bothering him or her. If you can help your child to figure out what is really wrong and meet the TRUE NEED of the emotion, then the eating disorder is obsolete. HOWEVER, you have to remember a very important point. Your child is not good at connecting feelings to life events, while they are VERY GOOD at responding to eating disorder related things. Thus, when they are at the top of the EATING DISORDER WAVE, they will associate their heightened intensity with the ED related event: NOT the REAL problem. Look at the difference between EMOTIONAL VENTING and EATING DISORDER VENTING.

TIP BOX

What are some things the Eating Disorder Filter concentrates on?
How full your child feels
How thing other people are
How clothes fit
Weight
Mirrors
Reflections in Windows
Calories in food
Calories being burned through exercise

For now, it is important to understand that when the eating disorder is loud in your child's head, she is at the TOP of the emotional wave. This is a very unstable place to be. ALSO IMPORTANT TO KNOW: NO LOGIC LIVES AT THE TOP OF THE WAVE. THUS TRYING TO TALK ABOUT THE ILLOGICAL NATURE OF EATING DISORDER

SPEAK WILL JUST MAKE THINGS WORSE! What is needed is for you to remain on the beach and help your child come down from the wave. Unfortunately, many parents go to the top of the wave instead!

It's peaceful down here. You can think clearly and solve problems down here. Bring your child down to you. Don't go up there and join her!

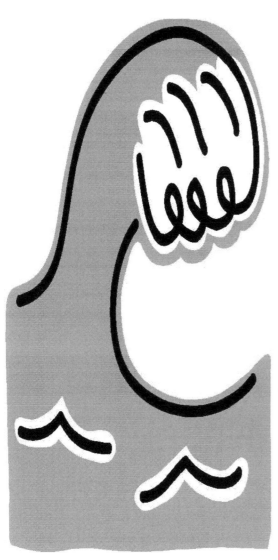

You are on the beach. Just revel in it!

You are at the top of the Eating Disorder Wave

Your EATING DISORDER IS SCREAMING OR YOU ARE VERY UPSET. You cannot think clearly when your emotions are this strong. You first need to use skills to calm down so that you can think clearly. Distraction and calming strategies would be helpful here. Then you can decide what to do. WHAT NOT TO DO: Don't be tricked by EATING DISORDER MIND. It knows you are upset and will try talking you into listening to it.

**What NOT to do:
ACT or LISTEN TO EATING DISORER MIND.
Don't act if you can't think.**

Your EATING DISORDER MIND is VERY LOUD. Your level of emotional energy is almost maxed out. It is difficult to think clearly here so you do not want to be thinking through solutions to your problems or giving others advice here. You may have a hard time using strategies to calm yourself down that require concentration (e.g. reading, word puzzles). You may have better luck with things that ABRUPTLY snap you out of it (driving and playing really loud music – blues preferred, a comedian on TV, a really HOT shower..). When you have regained some clarity, time to think!

**As your EATING DISORDER VOLUME goes up,
use strategies that require less concentration.**

Your EATING DISORDER MIND IS LOUD, but you can separate wisdom from EATING DISORDER MIND. Your level of emotional energy is definitely up, although you still have the ability to concentrate. A wide range of strategies could be used here: distraction, relaxation, etc. Check in with yourself to see if you REALLY can look at the situation without your emotions biasing what you see. If you can be objective, go into problem-solving mode. If not, stick with a distraction strategy a while longer. Emotion regulation sometimes takes a bit.

The lower your emotional intensity, the more options are available to you. Careful though. Don't go into "problem solving" until you REALLY have mental clarity.

EATING DISORDER MIND is pecking at you, but it is manageable. You notice your level of emotional energy starting to rise. Good for you! You have complete clarity and can do some self-coaching to figure out why you might be upset. Separate those aspects of the situation you have control over versus the aspects you need to work to accept. Make a plan to address the aspects you can affect. Use your wave skills to help tolerate the negative feelings that arise from accepting the aspects you can't do anything about.

Good problem solving involves separating the aspects of a situation you have control over from those you don't. You make a plan to address the aspects you can influence. You work on accepting the aspects you don't.

TIP BOX

Helping Your Child Off the Wave

What NOT to say: "Honey, you are on the wave. You really should go use some of the skills you learned at the doctor's office.

What to do INSTEAD: Join your child at the top of the wave (FIGURATIVELY, NOT LITERALLY) and practice using a strategy with him.

"You know what? You and I are both really upset right now. Let's leave the table and go for a walk around the block and then try again."

Works much better.   You'll see.

Key Points

o   Nobody thinks clearly when they are upset. Nobody. Get off the wave before you act.

o   Practicing good emotion regulation is important for several reasons: it provides a healthy example for your child and doesn't strengthen the eating disorder.

o   Your child's wave is a bit more complicated than yours because her or his emotional wave has the EATING DISORDER filter on top! Thus, whereas you may vent when you are upset, you are likely to hear "EATING DISORDER SPEAK" when your child is upset.

o   Logic doesn't work well with EATING DISORDER SPEAK. Instead, guide your child in the use of a coping strategy so you both are thinking more clearly.

Weekly Goals

Stay off the W.A.V.E. and think about a MASSAGE!!

Questions and Answers

Q: What if I manage my emotions very well, but it is my partner who is the problem? His/her temper with my child is really making things worse for our child.

A: This is an excellent, but tough, question. First, remember our golden rule. You can't control the emotions of others. You can just increase the likelihood they will be effective. Ultimately, they decide.

With that said, here are a few pointers.

Actually, the same strategies that work with a child work with a partner, a friend – you name it!

What NOT to do:

Inform your partner that he or she is losing their cool and needs to do something differently. FRUSTRATING for them.

What TO do (just a few suggestions, you may have developed much better strategies that work for you):

1. Put yourself in your partner's place and role model the use of a strategy (this is a bit sneaky). "Look honey, I am really upset right now and am afraid I'll say something I'll regret, I am going to go sit outside for a bit…"
2. Use compliments and positive strokes whenever you see the teeniest sign of effective behavior on the part of your partner. As you will learn in later sections, applying praise to baby steps will greatly increase the likelihood of future steps in the same direction!

Wisdom of the Week: My Gift to Myself

Have you taken our advice literally and really made a place for yourself in your home to relax and unwind? A place that is designated as YOURS and that no one is to BOTHER you if you go there unless there is a FIRE? I can't express how important it is to know you have a resting place. I would lose my mind if I didn't have one. In fact, children often recognize the need for this better than adults. Many children create secret hiding places that no one knows about. Smart little fellas. Think about it.

Date:

Remember our key guidelines

It's a process! Try, tweak, grow and learn.

Self-parenting: a necessary prerequisite for other parenting.

Learn how to SURF The WAVE!

Remain genuine.

Unhealthy or unhelpful behavior I will discuss WITH my child this week and our plan to address it.

Eats too little	Eats too little variety	Exercises too much
Throws up after meals	Doesn't get enough sleep	Doesn't set limits
Abuses laxatives	Engages in self-harm	Other

Possible Suggestions of How to Address:

☐ Ignore it

☐ Have a discussion about needed change in behavior
  *(discuss a future, necessary, logical consequence
  given the severity of the behavior)*

☐ Implement a logical consequence (reminding your
  child of the importance of health before anything)

☐ Appeal to your child's inner wisdom (have a discussion with your child about what you have observed,
  why you are concerned, the change in behavior
  expected)

☐ Reverse Time-Out (you leave)

☐ Group Time-Out (everyone leaves for 10 minutes)

☐ Regrouping (family meeting to get out of power
  struggle)

☐ Humor

My Plan:

Would a discussion be a good idea?

Heathy Coping Strategy I will address with my child this week and my plan to address it.

Express negative emotions effectively	Ask for more help	Set more limits (cut down study time, set a regular bedtime, cut out an activity)
Express an opinion- even if someone may disagree	Be more considerate of others	Place more realistic demands on oneself (consider the cost, not whether the demands are achieved)
Get a better balance of work and leisure	View a situation with curiosity rather than with criticism	Manage disappointing results
Share a vulnerability with someone	Embrace and learn from mistakes rather than running from them	Resolve a conflict
Tune in and respond more to what your feelings are telling you	Take more pride in oneself (being a more respectful self-parent)	Strut
Be Silly or just take yourself less seriously	Smile at your reflection	Initiate plans
Try something new	Get Messy	Break a ritual
Get more sleep	Other	Other

Possible Suggestions:	My Plan:
☐ Positive attention when takes a step toward behavior ☐ One-on-one time outside of eating disorder stuff ☐ Earning a logical privilege given increased health ☐ Praise and STOP – no BUTS ☐ Role Model Behavior Yourself ☐ Open the door for a discussion ☐ Set a limit ☐ Offer to teach ☐ Other	

Heathy Coping Strategy I will Role Model this week.

Possible Suggestions:	My Plan:
☐ Delegate something. ☐ Say 'no' to some things. ☐ Be honest with my feelings. ☐ Express my feelings when not on the wave. ☐ Ask for help. ☐ Set healthy limits between my needs and those of others. ☐ Listen with full attention. ☐ Praise and STOP. ☐ Say "I'm sorry" with no excuses. ☐ Allow family members to make mistakes without jumping in. ☐ Be consistent. ☐ Address negative self-talk. ☐ Be reliable.	

Self-care Strategy I will implement this week

Possible Suggestions:	My Plan:
☐ Make regular mealtimes a priority. ☐ Set a regular bedtime. ☐ Learn a new hobby. ☐ Spend some time with my friends. ☐ Spend time ALONE with my spouse. ☐ Set a regular time I stop work each day. ☐ Take weekends off. ☐ Buy something for myself. ☐ Exercise in a MODERATE manner. ☐ Take pride in my physical appearance.	No lame excuses!!

TIP OF THE WEEK: Put yourself in their shoes – for a moment.

CHAPTER FOUR: Strengthening Your Team

Where You Are

- ✓ You have finished your first step. You have learned more about the program.

- ✓ You have learned more about the stages of parenting and how eating disorders take your child off the path of healthy growth.

- ✓ You have learned a general approach to eating disorder management.

- ✓ You have learned how eating disorders serve as coping strategies.

- ✓ You have begun to get an idea of the targets you need to work on and have mobilized your family to start tackling these goals one at a time.

- ✓ You are beginning to appreciate the importance of yourself as a role model.

- ✓ You have learned how to maintain a clear mind by keeping your emotions at a level you can handle.

Congratulations.

Topic: Strengthening Your Team

In this section, our focus is on making sure YOU feel supported by loved ones, that you have helpers in place if you get upset and feel like "venting" to someone, and that you have people to call to run an errand if the demands of your child's illness make you feel paralyzed. After that introduction, many parents have the urge to skip this chapter and go on to the next chapter. *(Note: this urge usually occurs following the thought: "I can handle this. This doesn't apply to me. I don't want to burden anyone else with this; or, have people thinking I am a failure because my child has an eating disorder").* All I can say is: **please don't.** If I had a dime for every time a parent tried to convince me of the importance of managing this on his or her own.....and then have that same person say how much more meaningful their life has become because they got better at reaching out to others....I could retire.

Reaching out to others is important for a number of reasons:

> ~ You are acting as a healthy role model for your child, as asking for help is probably not one of his or her specialties.
> ~ It enables you to manage your child's illness, your own mental health, and your family more effectively.
> ~ It prevents burnout.
> ~ It decreases feelings of loneliness.
> ~ It helps to decrease the stigma of mental illness.

There are two traps I see parents fall into. We need to try to work through these traps because they may make managing your child's illness more difficult.

Trap #1 You keep your child's illness a SECRET from EVERYONE. Parents keep their child's illness a secret with very good intentions. They want to respect their child's privacy. They feel guilty or feel they have failed as parents and are embarrassed to tell others of their "perceived failures." They dread the unsolicited advice of family members who always seem to know everything. Those are all legitimate complaints. However, in my years of working with families, I have not seen these fears realized. Education of friends and family members helps people who care for you understand the difficulty of what you are going through. Information can help friends and family to be more understanding toward your child, and can help you feel less guilty. It also stops the "advice giving" because they begin to gain an understanding of how difficult this situation is.

In this chapter, we have you complete a social support activity. The purpose of this activity is for you to think about your different sources of support, to assess areas of weakness, and to THINK about who may be useful to talk to about your child's illness. This will lead to a helpful activity: discussing with your child your need to share your family's struggle with a FEW SPECIAL PEOPLE. More on this after you have completed the activity.

Trap #2 You don't involve your spouse or significant other because you don't want to burden him or her. This is really not a good idea. It communicates to your child that his or her problems are not significant or important enough to involve both parents. It makes your spouse or significant other feel unimportant.

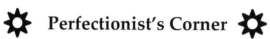

✿ Perfectionist's Corner ✿

<u>Perfectionist</u>:   But I don't like to make mistakes. I am not comfortable letting others know my family's problems. I feel bad enough that my child has an eating disorder. I don't want to share my problems with others – even if they are going through the same problem or have had the same problem in the past.

<u>Voice of Reason</u>: Whoa there! Let's take each of these protests, one at a time.

1. **First of all, there are NO MISTAKES in this program. In fact, there are NO MISTAKES outside of this program.**
   There is only growth from experiences. We experience things. We learn what works. We learn what doesn't. We tweak our behavior based on what we learn. That's all.

2. **Nobody is perfect.**
   Hard as it is to believe, even us psychologists misstep with our children and need to tweak our approach.   We are even totally inappropriate at times. We just have the curse of knowing we are doing it while we are doing it!

3. **Perfectionism can actually distance you from others.**
   Sadly, while many "perfectionists" fear that others will reject them for their flaws, the exact opposite is true. Acknowledging one's weaknesses is an important strength.   It shows we are genuine. It shows others we trust them enough to share this personal information. The opposite, i.e. refusing to acknowledge previous missteps, is distancing because others know that is just not true. Every one missteps. It is the wise ones, however, who are willing to try a different dance routine.

4. **People feel special when they are asked for help.**
   O.K. fine. I am a psychologist so I am going to be a bit biased about this. But it's true. Think how you feel when someone confides in you and asks your assistance. It's a compliment, isn't it? Does it make you feel trusted? And important?

5. **You are not a mind reader.**
   People have different limits. People also have different limits at different times. Sometimes they have all the energy and time in the world. Sometimes they feel

stretched in a million different directions. There is no way to know what a person's limits are at a certain time. They don't wear a sign on their foreheads that says, "I am really stretched to the limit right now. Please don't ask me to do anything." Importantly and fortunately, reading the limits of others is not your job. It is THEIR JOB to communicate them. Friendships and relationships go something like this:

Someone asks for assistance.

The other person helps if they can.

If they can't, they say so and the person who asks accepts their limits.

Then, when the other person needs help, the roles are reversed.

Dealing with "Well-Intended" but "Unhelpful" Advice from Others

Many families I work with struggle with how to manage the advice from friends, family and, particularly, their own parents. In fact, I have a rule I often tell these families:

> "Imagine the stupidest thing a family member can say.
> Bet money they will say it. You will not be disappointed."

For many reasons (which I will explain), people who care about us love to give us advice, even when we haven't asked for it (hmm, sound familiar). They do this for many good reasons:

1. They may hate to see you in pain and want to do anything in their power to reduce your pain.
2. They feel powerless and it is the only thing they can think to do – run at the mouth.
3. They are terrified the same thing will happen to their child so they try to offer simple solutions in the hopes that the problem is simple.
4. They lack confidence in their own parenting and thus giving others advice makes them feel better about themselves (sadly, often at others' expense).

Although hearing such advice can be hard, it is actually an excellent opportunity to role model some very important things for your child: making the opinions of others not matter so much in determining your value as a person.

The opinions of others are only as important as you make them.
Chances are, your child struggles greatly with placing too much emphasis on the opinions of others. This is not a healthy way to be because we can't control the opinions of others. Thus, if our self-esteem depends on others liking us, we are in a very vulnerable position as some people will like us, some won't; some will like us on some days, some on others – you get the picture. If, instead, our opinion of ourselves is based on the self-respect and self-regard in which we hold ourselves, we are in GREAT SHAPE, as we TOTALLY CONTROL that!

You know what Self? I really like you. I don't care what anyone else things. If they don't like me or approve of my parenting, they are missing out on a charming individual.

Fortunately or unfortunately, the world is what it is. We can't make the world safe and we can't make people say the right things. Instead, we have to help our children (and ourselves) cope with what's out there. When you take that perspective, life becomes a lot less threatening. Remember my analogy early in the first chapter (of course you do). If life is a river, then we can learn to become better navigators so we are able to handle any turn in the journey. Instead, very anxious people try to control which way the river will go; a losing proposition.

It might also help to think back to the last time you had the urge to give someone advice on something – how to get along with a difficult coworker or how to get their son to bed on time – and think back to your reasons in doing so. Maybe you didn't want to see your friend struggle, or maybe it felt good to offer a helpful suggestion. Chances are you didn't walk away thinking to yourself that your friend was a disaster in the workplace or as a parent. But sometimes we really do just need someone to listen, and it might be helpful to give your friends a heads up that this is what you're looking for, when you just need some time to vent.

TIP BOX

In terms of stupid comments, you have a number of options.

Your relative: "Oh my goodness. Your daughter is so thin. I would never let my daughter get that thin. My daughter and I have a very close relationship. How did you let that happen?"

1. Ignore them. You: "Have you finished your holiday shopping yet? I have been shopping online. What a lifesaver! I'm finished already.

2. Be catty in your mind. You (in your mind): "Yes, and I am sure your daughter will really enjoy it when you insist on going with her on her honeymoon.

3. Educate them. You: "You're telling me. If someone would have told me a year ago that my family would go through this, I would have never believed them. I wouldn't wish this on anyone, but I will say that my family has gotten so much closer and stronger as a result of this experience."

4. Be a smart aleck. You: "Well, actually, I have been planning this for years. I thought to myself, 'Now, how can I make sure that my child develops an eating disorder? Let me make sure that I make that happen.'"

What about the siblings?

Parents struggle a great deal with how to protect their other children from the impact of the Eating Disorder. I want to share with you what works.

What Works
1. Don't keep your children in the dark. Educate them about their sibling's illness (ideally in the presence of their sibling – this works best if your child explains things to his siblings).
2. Keep the siblings talking: have the child with the eating disorder tell his or her siblings how they can be helpful; have the siblings share how the eating disorder is interfering with healthy family life. **Work as a team to take steps towards health while your family minimizes the impact of the eating disorder on the family.** REACH A COMPROMISE BETWEEN THE TWO POSITIONS.
3. When your child with an eating disorder asks her siblings for help, make sure s/he is speaking from a place of wisdom and not on top of the Eating Disorder Wave. **Fair Request: Could the family please stop talking about weight and dieting during mealtimes? Unfair Request: Could you please only keep low-calorie products in the house? Fair Request: Could you not leave cookies on the counter because I don't feel safe not to binge on them? Unfair Request: Could you never talk about snack foods again?**
4. The job of your other children is to support their sibling and provide encouragement. **Your other children are not to be the food police. Not ever. Way too much pressure. Their job is to cheerlead. Only.**
5. Ask your other children for help with OTHER things. Although, your children should not be the food police, they can be very helpful with picking up some extra chores around the house given all the traveling you have to do, getting dinner started, arranging car pools, etc.

Section Activity: Figuring out Your Social Support Network.

Take a look at the following diagram and definitions on the following page. In each circle, write down who currently fits in that definition. Following that, answer the questions. Please.

Use the following definitions to fill in your circles on the next page.

My Inner Circle.

These are very special people. They know just about everything about you – and they like you anyways ☺. You would not think twice about asking them for help in a time of emergency because that is the type of relationship you have. You would do the same for them. If you are rude to each other, you feel very comfortable letting the other person know your feelings. These are people you have CLOSE, GENUINE, relationships with. SPECIAL, SPECIAL PEOPLE.

My Middle Circle.

These are good friends. They know a lot about you. For example, they probably know a great deal about your day-to-day activities and stressors. They may not know very intimate details about your history, but they might. You look forward to spending time with them. You share things with them. You look to them for instrumental support (they would certainly do you a favor, but you would be inclined to make sure you return the favor in kind).

My Outer Circle.

These are casual friends. You are friendly to them. It is nice to see them. You probably don't go out of your way to make plans with them other than during the context in which your path's cross. You enjoy their company. They probably know the members of your family and relevant details; however, you would not ask them for things outside of the context in which your path's cross. For example, if you knew them at work, you may ask them to cover your job and make arrangement to cover their job in the future.

Using these as guidelines, fill in the circles below.

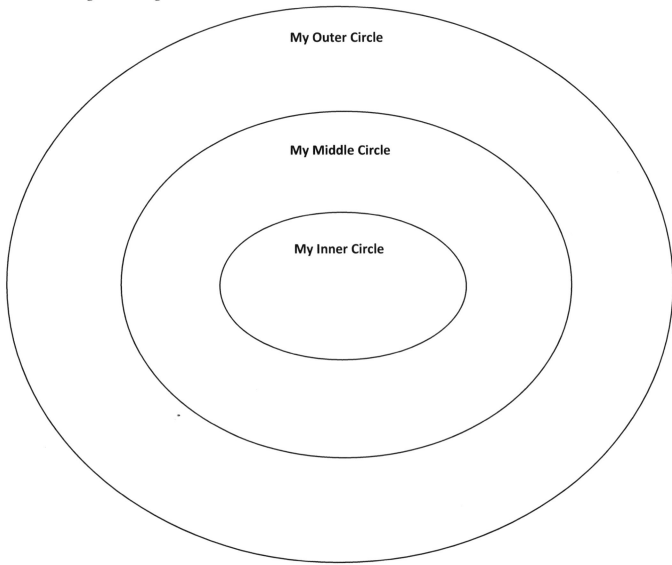

Examining Your Circles

Take a look at what you wrote down and answer the following questions (not in your head!) Go ahead a write down the answers. This makes you think about it more.

1. Take a look at your inner circle. Are there people in your inner circle? Are there any people in your middle circle that have the potential to become insiders? If so, what are some things you are willing to share with these individuals to bring them one step closer?

2. Take a look at your outer circle. Are there any people in your outer circle that have the potential to become middlers? If so, what are some things you are willing to share with these individuals to bring them one step closer? What are you willing to do with these people to bring them one step closer?

3. Think about your relationship with yourself. Where would you put yourself? Are you a member of your own inner circle? If not, what are some kind and gentle things you can for yourself to bring yourself one step closer to your heart?

4. If you are involved in a significant, intimate relationship, is that person a member of your inner circle? If not, why not?

5. Are your parents members of the inner circle? If not, why not? Is this a relationship worth working on? What can you do?

TIP BOX: Tending to Our Relationships

What does it take to be a good friend or a good companion?   The following suggestions are adapted from the wonderful writings and research of a colleague of mine, Steven Asher of Duke University, who specializes in the study of childhood friendship formation (however, the same rules apply to adults)!

1. You initiate plans with people outside of situations in which you ordinarily run into them.

It's one thing to have lunch with colleagues at work. However, it takes the relationship one big step closer when you initiate plans with this person – call them on the phone to see how they are doing, invite them over, go to a movie with them, etc. When someone does this to you, doesn't it make you feel special? Sure it does! It shows how much they enjoy your company.

2. You can share in their accomplishments and be accepting of their flaws.

Friends are not competitors. Friends share in the joy of one another's accomplishments or are genuine enough that they can be honest about their own insecurities and feelings of jealousy. Friends remain friends even after one member has revealed a flaw. The relationship would be very unstable if this were not the case, wouldn't it?

3. You attend to conflicts.

Friends have disagreements. People in intimate relationship have disagreements. Families have disagreements. Quality relationships demand that people discuss what happened, take ownership of what they can do differently next time, and move on.

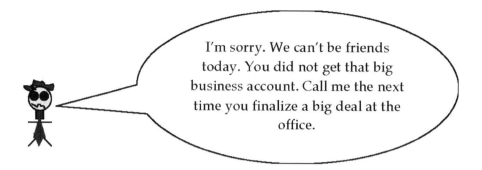

I'm sorry. We can't be friends today. You did not get that big business account. Call me the next time you finalize a big deal at the office.

TIP BOX (continued)

4. You are reliable.

You know our motto: Do what you say and say what you mean.

5. You know how to share: time, opinions, feelings, faults...

Think balance: your interests with their interests, listening and talking, sharing and supporting. Relationships are yet another great example of the dance: a quality relationship has a lovely rhythm to it.

6. You are genuine.

Relationships are about honesty. Good relationships require you to be honest about your opinions and feelings – even if it hurts the other person's feelings sometimes. To do otherwise is to have a very superficial relationship.

7. You set limits when you need to.

Sometimes we just can't help our friends or partners when he or she needs us to. Life is what it is. We do what we can and are comfortable saying no when we have to.

Key Points

- Asking for help from others is important to preserve your mental health, to prevent burnout, and to set a good example.
- Needing others brings people closer and demonstrates our humanness.
- If possible, both parents need to be involved. There are always exceptions, but unacceptable excuses are:
  - Work schedule won't permit.
  - I don't want to burden him or her.
  - That would interfere with the racket ball season.

Weekly Goals

- Complete your social support activity (if you haven't already).
- Have a discussion with your child about sharing what is going on with close friends and family.
- Reach out to someone.
- Do something supportive for yourself.

Questions and Answers

Q: I have several children. How can I involve my spouse when someone has to care for the children?

A: An eating disorder is a family problem. As a family, it is important to discuss what is going on with your child and how everyone can support your child getting help. When one family member is in trouble, the family needs to work together to make sure the illness gets targeted; yet, that the illness does not run the family. We'll explain this more in the next chapter. In brief, the family supports behaviors towards health in all of its members but does not support behaviors that prolong illness. Treatment is good, so the family mobilizes to make sure treatment can happen. It can be challenging to juggle all of your regular work and family responsibilities in addition to appointments with doctors and clinicians. This may be a time when your family needs additional support from friends and family, so that both you and your spouse can participate in this process.

Q: I am a very private person. I am just not comfortable talking to others about my problems.

A: Thanks for being honest about your struggles. When you go to your chair after reading this, I want you to think about the barriers that make it hard for you to share. Maybe you have been taught that asking for help is a sign of weakness? Maybe you don't want to burden others with your struggle? Think for a moment how you feel when someone comes to you with their troubles and asks you for support or advice. Makes you feel important and trusted, doesn't it? Asking for help is a balancing act, a dance between people. We have to balance meeting our own needs with asking. It is not our job to anticipate or mind read how much help is appropriate. Rather, it is other peoples' job to communicate their personal boundaries so we know when we are asking for too much.

Q: My other children are feeling neglected.

A: This is a tough one! Managing an entire family when one member has a serious illness is terribly difficult. One idea we have seen families use very effectively is creating new family rituals. The problem of sharing parents' time among many siblings is one every family must face, whether or not one of them has an illness. We have seen some parents create a special time for each child each week or every other week that is reserved for just that child. It is important that this be a scheduled time for you and your child and that you schedule other things around this time, as you would for every other important appointment you have. For example, my father and I would always go out to breakfast, just the two of us, one morning every week. This was exceedingly special to me as it indicated to me that I was important enough that my dad wanted to spend time with me. I shall always remember that time.

Q: I want to seek support from friends, but I don't want to burden them. How do I know when it is too much?

I want to remind you about a point that was made earlier in this chapter (that I am sure you have not forgotten already!). You are NOT a mind reader. Thus, you can have no idea what is a burden for your friend. It is your friend's job to tell you that; you can't be expected to guess. Some of the parents I work with have an easier time asking if they say something related to that first. For example, you might say, "I am going to trust you to be honest with me if something I am asking you to do is too much and to trust that I will totally understand. Deal?" Deal.

Wisdom of the Week: My Gift to Myself

Go on a date. If you are married, how about your spouse? If not married, how about a close friend? Or, if you desperately need alone time, how about a date with yourself?

Date:

Remember our key guidelines

It's a process! Try, tweak, grow and learn.

Self-parenting: a necessary prerequisite for other parenting.

Learn how to SURF The WAVE!

Remain genuine.

Unhealthy or unhelpful behavior I will discuss WITH my child this week and our plan to address it.

Eats too little	Eats too little variety	Exercises too much
Throws up after meals	Doesn't get enough sleep	Doesn't set limits
Abuses laxatives	Engages in self-harm	Other

Possible Suggestions of How to Address:

☐ Ignore it

☐ Have a discussion about needed change in behavior *(discuss a future, necessary, logical consequence given the severity of the behavior)*

☐ Implement a logical consequence (reminding your child of the importance of health before anything)

☐ Appeal to your child's inner wisdom (have a discussion with your child about what you have observed, why you are concerned, the change in behavior expected)

☐ Reverse Time-Out (you leave)

☐ Group Time-Out (everyone leaves for 10 minutes)

☐ Regrouping (family meeting to get out of power struggle)

☐ Humor

My Plan:

Would a discussion be a good idea?

Heathy Coping Strategy I will address with my child this week and my plan to address it.

Express negative emotions effectively	Ask for more help	Set more limits (cut down study time, set a regular bedtime, cut out an activity)
Express an opinion- even if someone may disagree	Be more considerate of others	Place more realistic demands on oneself (consider the cost, not whether the demands are achieved)
Get a better balance of work and leisure	View a situation with curiosity rather than with criticism	Manage disappointing results
Share a vulnerability with someone	Embrace and learn from mistakes rather than running from them	Resolve a conflict
Tune in and respond more to what your feelings are telling you	Take more pride in oneself (being a more respectful self-parent)	Strut
Be Silly or just take yourself less seriously	Smile at your reflection	Initiate plans
Try something new	Get Messy	Break a ritual
Get more sleep	Other	Other

Possible Suggestions:	**My Plan:**
☐ Positive attention when takes a step toward behavior ☐ One-on-one time outside of eating disorder stuff ☐ Earning a logical privilege given increased health ☐ Praise and STOP – no BUTS ☐ Role Model Behavior Yourself ☐ Open the door for a discussion ☐ Set a limit ☐ Offer to teach ☐ Other	

Heathy Coping Strategy I will Role Model this week.

Possible Suggestions:	**My Plan:**
☐ Delegate something. ☐ Say 'no' to some things. ☐ Be honest with my feelings. ☐ Express my feelings when not on the wave. ☐ Ask for help. ☐ Set healthy limits between my needs and those of others. ☐ Listen with full attention. ☐ Praise and STOP. ☐ Say "I'm sorry" with no excuses. ☐ Allow family members to make mistakes without jumping in. ☐ Be consistent. ☐ Address negative self-talk. ☐ Be reliable.	

Self-care Strategy I will implement this week

Possible Suggestions:	**My Plan:**
☐ Make regular mealtimes a priority. ☐ Set a regular bedtime. ☐ Learn a new hobby. ☐ Spend some time with my friends. ☐ Spend time ALONE with my spouse. ☐ Set a regular time I stop work each day. ☐ Take weekends off. ☐ Buy something for myself. ☐ Exercise in a MODERATE manner. ☐ Take pride in my physical appearance.	No lame excuses!!

TIP OF THE WEEK: Bring yourself to Your Inner Circle.

CHAPTER FIVE: Ins and Outs of Healthy Eating

Where You Are

- ✓ You have finished your first step.   You have learned more about the program.

- ✓ You have learned more about the stages of parenting and how eating disorders take your child off the path of healthy growth.

- ✓ You have learned a general approach to eating disorder management.

- ✓ You have learned how eating disorders serve as coping strategies.

- ✓ You have begun to get an idea of the targets you need to work on and have mobilized your family to start tackling these goals one at a time.

- ✓ You are beginning to appreciate the importance of yourself as a role model.

- ✓ You have learned how to maintain a clear mind by keeping your emotions at a level you can handle.

- ✓ You have gathered a loyal team of supporters.

Congratulations.

Topic: Healthy Eating

This chapter focuses on the steps your child will progress through regarding the restoration of healthy eating. First, we take a trip back to remember what healthy eating looks like from childhood to adulthood. Next, we introduce the eating disorder into this sequence and discuss some of the traps that get in the way of this process.

> Well, this has nothing to do with my eating disorder, but I have decided to become a lacto-super-duper-ovo-feminist-kosher, anti-oxidant eater. Basically, I will not eat anything from a factory that employs females in inferior positions to men, does not follow orthodox dietary rules, will avoid animal and dairy foods, will not eat vegetables from the same farm as ....

A Friendly Reminder of Healthy Eating: Teamwork Through the Ages

Eating disorders often cause parents to lose their footing regarding how to nourish their children. Because of this, it's helpful to think about what healthy looks like so we can gain a reasonable perspective regarding your family's eating environment.

The Younger Years

When your children are children, the roles of parents in relation to their children's meals are pretty straightforward. Parents plan the meals and establish regular meal and snack times. They purchase and prepare the food. Your child's job is to perform his or her chores in relation to mealtimes (setting the table, clearing, sweeping, washing dishes -whatever the rules are in your house), to be in attendance at family meals (more about this in a later chapter), to behave respectfully at the dinner table, and to eat FROM WHAT IS SERVED. This last point could use some elaboration. Imagine your child is going to a dinner party at another person's house. Would you ever want this to happen?

> Uh, excuse me, Mrs. Friendly Neighbor.
> Thank you so much for inviting me over for dinner.
> I actually do not like what you have made.
> Can you please make me something else?

Of course not! You would be mortified. The same behavior should be expected at your home. You make a meal and your child eats from what is served. They don't have to eat the parts they don't like, and you, being a respectful parent, try to have at least a few parts of the meal that your whole family likes. However, family members need to be courteous in their refusal. Meals are about BALANCE; balancing food groups, balancing new foods with familiar foods, etc…

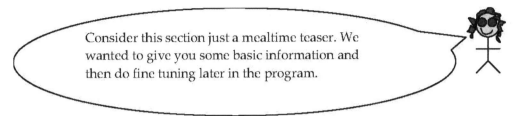

Consider this section just a mealtime teaser. We wanted to give you some basic information and then do fine tuning later in the program.

Younger and Middle Adolescence

Eating disorder or no eating disorder, a lot of families seem to lose their footing during this period. I'll tell you what IS HEALTHY. Families should KEEP HAVING FAMILY MEALS - AS OFTEN AS POSSIBLE. This is one of the greatest tragedies of modern life -that we are losing this sacred tradition. I feel so strongly about this that I devote an entire chapter to it, so I won't go into a lot of depth here. For now, just keep the take home point: family meals are always important, even when your child behaves as if you are the least important thing to do on a list of important things to do!

What does change regarding healthy eating during adolescence? Well, several things. First, your child can do more so that means they can help more. They can help make dinners. They can have increased input on the menu. The older they get, the more their input is valued and incorporated. I know some families in which every member plans a dinner, trades off helping, whatever. However, the same rules as above apply.

TIP BOX

The Expectations of Healthy Children at Mealtimes

    ~ Be present frequently

    ~ Contribute as part of the family team

    ~ Eat from what is served

    ~ Be polite

Not rocket science – just reasonable expectations. If they don't like the entrée, they can eat the sides; however, NOT LIKING the entrée doesn't excuse them from the meal. Their company is valued no matter what.

So what about adolescent food quirks or dieting or whatever? Well, I'll speak a bit about healthy nutrition, but really the same spirit applies: **discussion and compromise.** If a family member has an important moral belief concerning food (e.g. vegetarianism) that is rooted in health, you stick to our magic formula of discussion and reasonable compromise and come up with a solution that respects your child's individuality while not inconveniencing the rest of the family. Maybe your child will add the vegetarian side dish; maybe vegetarian entrees will alternate with meat, etc.

Adult Children

As you may have surmised by now, the SPIRIT of the principles don't change very much when your child is an adult. Communication, courtesy, and wisdom are always key. However, if your adult child is living in your home, there is a need to clearly delineate expectations and to define courtesy. There is no one right way – any way can work provided it is a discussion guided by mutual respect. Things that need discussion when you have an adult child living in your home:

- Expectations regarding attendance at meals
- Expectations regarding notification about not attending meals (it's rude for your child to not show up for dinner when she or he is expected)
- Expectations regarding contributions to meals

What many parents with an adult child living in their home would like to say…

You are an adult. When I was your age, I expected NOTHING from my parents and was already holding down three jobs and raising 20 kids. The LEAST you can do since we are good enough to continue to let you live here when, in fact, we were looking forward to having no kids at home, is to take the trouble to CALL if you are not coming for dinner, or take out the trash every once in a while.

What many parents with an adult child living in their home could say…

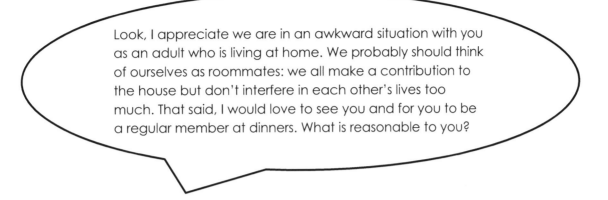

Look, I appreciate we are in an awkward situation with you as an adult who is living at home. We probably should think of ourselves as roommates: we all make a contribution to the house but don't interfere in each other's lives too much. That said, I would love to see you and for you to be a regular member at dinners. What is reasonable to you?

A Friendly Reminder of Healthy Eating: The Food

You get the gist: discussion, team-work, mutual respect, and courtesy are the keys to healthy mealtime interactions. What about the food? I've got key words for this as well: balance, moderation, variety, and common sense.

Balance
Think of two teeter-totters crossing. Balance is about having some "weight" on all the sides of the teeter totter so everyone is about the same height. There are several things to balance in meal planning: • Food groups (some bread products, some fruit, some vegetables, some dairy, some meat or meat substitute, some fat) • High fat balanced with low fat = a moderate amount of fat – think on average, not on each individual item! • New foods with familiar foods

What do you mean my fat-free, low-calorie mango salsa and rice cakes in not a balance meal?!! It's got mangos, onions, tomatoes,

Don't forget about the "common sense" part. That will usually save you at times like these.

Moderation
You know the saying: too much of a good thing…. By moderation we mean: • Listening to your body (when you are healthy) to help you to determine fullness • Balancing meal size throughout the day rather than saving it all up for the evening • Key to moderation: insert a pause between servings. Give yourself 5-10 minutes. Listen to your body. Still hungry? Take more.

> Wow, kids, that was impressive! You've eaten an entire meal in 30 seconds. This has been really enjoyable family time.

TIP BOX

By moderation, we mean respecting your body's cues of hunger and cues of fullness. To do this here are some tricks:

- Wait 5-10 minutes between helpings to make sure your body is telling for seconds and not your mind.

- Meals need to last at least 20 minutes for your mind to register fullness.

- Try to have meals last anywhere from 20-45 minutes to slow the pace and have good conversation.

> Uh, what should I do if my child takes 20 YEARS to eat a meal? It is driving me insane.

Tackle one thing at a time, and don't forget…discussion and compromise.

Variety

What is a healthy amount of variety? Although I know some of you black and white thinkers out there would love for me to give you a number, I can't. O.K. 20. This is where the common sense part comes in. We all get into food ruts at times. No big deal. The point of variety is that no food gives us everything we need so by balancing food groups and choosing some different foods within each group, you'll hit everything.

In each food group, some foods have greater **_nutrient density_** than others: i.e. more vitamins and minerals per calorie than others. Think of 1 cup of broccoli and 1/8 cup of jelly beans. Both of these foods have the same amount of energy (calories); however, it doesn't take too much thinking to realize that the broccoli gives you a lot more for your calories (fiber, vitamins, minerals, etc.) than the jelly beans.

There is another catch that we'll address in the TRAPS section. In each food group, some foods have more calories than others. If we have variety, sometimes we choose the higher, sometimes the lower and it all balances out. Your child will likely try to always shoot for the lower....variety protects against this.

Common Sense

Ah, common sense. The thing we seem to lose track of when we are dealing with an eating disorder. Eating in a healthy way in today's diet-obsessed world isn't easy – unless you fall back on common sense.

As consumers of food and diet products, we are the targets of more food marketing campaigns like never before. Sadly, ingenious marketing strategies are even being targeted to children, as children greatly influence the purchasing behavior of their parents and have more access to money of their own. Thus, our best strategy is to ROLE MODEL being a critical consumer and to TEACH being a critical consumer to our children.

Rather than go into a media literacy lesson, I will just emphasize some logical, basic principles. The diet industry is a billion dollar industry – ANNUALLY. On the reverse side, what I lovingly refer to as "crap food production" – chemicals thrown together, shaped, artificially colored and named "food" – continues to increase. To navigate these two extremes, stick to the basics.

Tip Box: The Basics

1. Restrictive diets or extreme diets that have people eliminate entire food groups don't work and don't make a lot of sense. If they did work, they wouldn't have to keep inventing new ones, would they? If you are moderately active, use balance, moderation, variety, and common sense and your body will take care of you. Each few years they switch the "bad" food group. They sell millions, we are suckers, and no one is better off. STAY MODERATE. Help your child and yourself avoid the hype.

2. Eat food – not a bunch of chemicals. When in doubt, look at the list of ingredients. Is anything recognizable? Is there any food in there? I am a believer in whole foods: foods that are natural and wholesome. Peanut butter crisp cereal, deep fried cupcakes, -"alleged foods" like that are a lot of things and some of these "alleged foods" are quite tasty, but they are not food. Eat mainly FOOD.

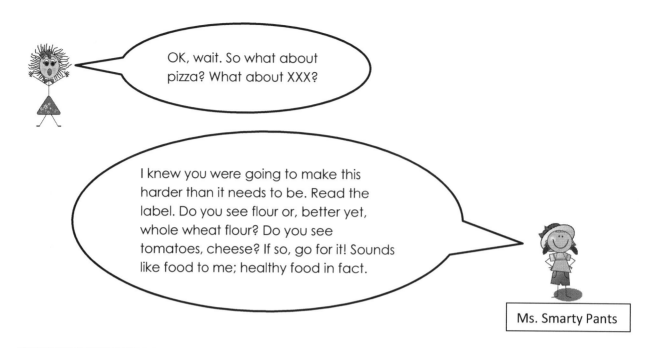

OK, wait. So what about pizza? What about XXX?

I knew you were going to make this harder than it needs to be. Read the label. Do you see flour or, better yet, whole wheat flour? Do you see tomatoes, cheese? If so, go for it! Sounds like food to me; healthy food in fact.

Ms. Smarty Pants

Tip Box: The Basics, cont'd

3.   Deprivation vs. respect is a matter of wisdom and semantics. Make healthy choices, not because certain food are "forbidden" or "evil" or because you "don't allow" yourself to have groups of chemicals thrown together, but because you respect your body and feel good when you eat well. You can if you want, and if you want, do so. Focus on how your body feels – not rigid rules.

4.   So, are there good foods and bad foods? C'mon. Give us the answer. You're killing me. No. Some foods are healthier than others. When people eat the amount of energy (in the form of calories) their body needs to maintain their weight, they will not gain weight, no matter how crappy the food. However, they won't be very healthy because they are not getting the vitamins and minerals they need.

5.   How often should you eat foods that are a bunch of chemicals thrown together? If you fit them in, you could have them every day. Focus on how your body feels. Say that again. To clarify….the new food guide pyramid put out by the United Stated Department of Agriculture has an interesting way of explaining this: DISCRETIONARY CALORIES. For each person's energy needs (which considers things like age, gender, and activity), they provide a "pyramid" – a list of servings from the food groups that provide the vitamins and minerals your body needs. Once you eat that, you have some calories "left over." You spend these how you want.

The Food: Putting It All Together

So, what do balance, moderation, variety, and common sense look like when you put it all together? Well, it might look like this:

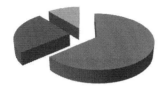

■ Low Risk   ■ Medium Risk   ■ High Risk

In addition, I asked a nutritionist at Duke to put together a sample menu of what a relatively active female adolescent would need to eat to MAINTAIN her weight. I wanted to include this to give you some perspective. Often the eating of an adolescent with an eating disorder has gotten so skewed over time that we have forgotten what healthy eating looks like. To repeat, this is what a healthy adolescent might eat if her weight WERE TO REMAIN THE SAME. To GAIN WEIGHT, a person needs to consume about 500 EXTRA CALORIES every day, IN ADDITION to what their body needs to maintain their weight. So, let's think of this person. This is a normal day of eating for this healthy, relatively active adolescent.

BALANCED MENUS FOR ACTIVE TEENS

Breakfast
Honey Nut Cheerios with low fat milk (or soy milk) and a small sliced banana
Scrambled egg
Cup of orange juice

Lunch
Sandwich: 2 slices whole grain bread, with 2 to 3 ounces of lean ham, slice of Swiss cheese, honey mustard and chopped lettuce
Carrot sticks with small amount of dressing to dip in
Fresh pear
Hershey kisses (4 or 5)
Water

Afternoon Snack
Crackers with peanut butter
Applesauce cup

Dinner
BBQ chicken breast
Small roasted potatoes, brushed with olive oil
Serving of green beans
Tossed salad with regular dressing
Small dinner roll Glass of skim or low fat milk (or soy milk)

Evening Snack
Frozen yogurt with granola topping

If we wanted this person to gain a pound in a week, s/he must add about 500 calories to what s/he is already eating. What are some things about equal to 500 calories??

- A bakery-sized whole wheat bagel with a few thumbs full of peanut butter
- 3 tennis-ball size servings of cereal with a cupcake wrapper size full of milk
- 2 tennis ball size bowls of granola
- A cupcake wrapper filled with nuts and a cupcake wrapper filled with raisins
- A slice of whole wheat pita bread with two large pieces of REAL cheese and a handful of pretzels

Just to give you an idea….

Nutrition Education 101 In Relation to Eating Disorders

Our goal is not to present you with basic nutrition education. There are many wonderful professional and government organizations that produce excellent publications on healthy eating. Instead, we'll focus on specific problems with nutrition in eating disorder management.

There is no one "right" way to nourish your child back to health.

Don't forget our refrain: you try something, you see how it works, you tweak it. You try again. That said, we can provide some helpful tricks we have found that moves things along.

First, it may be helpful to consider the way in which a nutritionist often goes about meal planning. S/he calculates a ROUGH estimate of the amount of nourishment your child needs to maintain a healthy weight (often using special formulas that consider, age, height, and level of activity). Then s/he considers the level of calories your child has been consuming. S/he then considers the discrepancy between these two places and makes a stepwise plan to bring the child's eating up to the level that is healthy.

Nutrition (calories) your child needs to eat for health
+ Amount of food your child is currently eating
= Amount needed to be increased for health

There are three factors that need to be addressed: 1) the amount of calories, 2) the food groups and balance those calories represent, and 3) the variety in the foods chosen. Because each of these issues may be fearful for your child, often they are done in a stepwise fashion with the increase in the AMOUNT of calories being the most important first step, balance second, and variety third. After your child has mastered, and feels comfortable with, the **mechanical aspects of eating ~ eating a healthy, balanced diet on a schedule ~ then we move on to training your child to be better attuned to his or her hunger cues and to use those cues to guide the amounts eaten at meals.**
Warning: expect these steps to move slowly…

Nutritional Needs are a Moving Target – Not an Exact, Stagnant Figure

To better understand body weight regulation, it is helpful to compare body weight to another fluctuating entity in our bodies: blood sugar.

Blood sugar is constantly fluctuating. When individuals with diabetes record their daily blood sugar throughout the day, they get a variety of different values – **even if they were to follow a prescribed diabetic diet to the letter.** Why? Well, the body is an amazingly complex machine and blood sugar is affected by many, many variables in your body, the majority of which are beyond an individual's PRECISE control. The behaviors an individual with diabetes has control over: healthy eating, moderate physical activity, taking medications, etc. maximize the LIKELIHOOD that their blood sugars will remain regulated but do not GUARANTEE it. We just don't have that kind of control. Thus, physicians and diabetes educators prescribe a certain level of medication or insulin and then modify that prescription based on the patient's subsequent blood sugar log.

Body weight regulation works in a similar fashion. The behaviors that we have "control" over, our healthy eating and exercise, increase the likelihood that we will regulate a healthy body weight but they don't guarantee it. Why? Well, because many variables affect our body weight regulation on a moment to moment basis: the amount of water in our body, our hormones, our body's electrolyte balance, and on and on. Thus, a body weight journal would look very similarly to a blood sugar journal – a lot of fluctuating values that vary around a constant range. Your children tend to get excessively agitated over the fluctuations and forget that we are looking at trends over time. Don't forget this: weight fluctuates, when there is a consistent trend of weight loss or weight gain, we consider that a true gain or loss.

Enter: The Eating Disorder and the Traps to Healthy Eating

So, now you understand what is supposed to happen during HEALTHY development and how to incorporate these principles to help your child. Despite this, there are some traps parents fall into that I will tell you about so you can be ready for them!

We'll explain this by highlighting some traps that often get in the way of nutrition and health in the context of eating disorders.

Trap #1: You are confused regarding who you are cooking for: your child's eating disorder, your child, or the rest of the family.

As with everything related to parenting, your role may vary depending both on your child's age and stage in the illness. Let's first remind you of our general stance towards parenting: the DANCE.

Tip Box: The Dance of Parenting

Remember when they were little? When teaching your child a new skill, you went through the dance of parenting without really thinking about it. Imagine you wanted to teach your child to tie her or his shoe. First, you showed him or her the steps to tying your shoe. Next, you tied your child's shoe with him or her. Then, you stepped back and allowed your child to try on his or her own. If you child struggled a little, you stayed back and let your child wrestle through and learn. If he or she was really struggling, you stepped in and helped some more. It is this back and forth of leaning in and stepping back that I refer to as the "dance" of parenting. You lose your rhythm when you are afraid to step back and give your child a try, and you lose your step when you don't lean in when they need you. Figuring this out is just a matter of trying different strategies and seeing what works. However, you have to try a strategy many times before you give up and try an alternative – just remember that.

Young children and young adolescents (roughly 3-14 years)

Enter an eating disorder. One goal of managing an eating disorder is maximizing your child's return to health while minimizing the impact of the illness on your child and the family. This is true regardless of your child's age. This brings us to two important questions:

1. Should the family eat what the child with the eating disorder eats?
2. Conversely, should the child with the eating disorder eat what the family eats?

Question 1. Should the family eat what the child with the eating disorder eats? Oh, no. That would be cruel. Have you seen some of the bizarre concoctions individuals with eating disorders come up with?

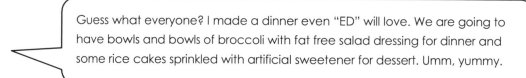

Guess what everyone? I made a dinner even "ED" will love. We are going to have bowls and bowls of broccoli with fat free salad dressing for dinner and some rice cakes sprinkled with artificial sweetener for dessert. Umm, yummy.

See what we mean? Often, eating disorder "safe" meals are not safe at all! They are not only unhealthy, but also lack much taste.

Question 2. Conversely, should the child with the eating disorder eat what the family eats? Yes and no. First, some background information. When someone is fearful of something and we are teaching skills so they can approach their fears, there are several steps involved. First, we have to teach them coping skills to manage the anxiety or fear that will occur when facing a fear. Second, we help the individual to approach fears in a very stepwise fashion: starting with smaller fears and working our way, bit by bit, up to larger fears. Thus, when we are working on restoring the nourishment of your child, we often start with increasing the amount of safe foods (foods your child can eat reasonably comfortably) and then by working with increased balance and variety.

Tip Box: Your Child's Fear of Out-of-Control Eating

I have many individuals I work with tell me that they are afraid of eating good tasting food because currently they eat large amounts of high-fiber, low-calorie foods and never get full. Well, there are several problems with this line of reasoning. Although low calorie foods that are high in fiber are filling in the short term (because they contain a lot of water and bulk), this feeling of fullness does not last long because your child is still not eating the amount of balanced ENERGY he/she needs. You need balance in the form of carbohydrate, protein, and fat to REMAIN satiated. Second, there are two types of satiety: physical fullness and TASTE satiety. True "satisfaction and fullness" requires that you satisfy both of these things. Thus, large amounts of tasteless food will not meet this requirement. Ironically, if your child allowed him/herself to eat tasty food regularly, he would get satisfied with less food.

In the beginning, if your child has been eating tasteless food and starts eating TASTY food, s/he may have the urge to eat more. Of course. It is novel and actually tastes good. In addition, he may fear that the eating disorder part of himself will take this food away and thus, he wants to eat as much as he can before the evil part of him stops him. By talking about these things and working as a team, you can help your child through all these fears.

Trap #2: You continue to compare your child's current eating to his other eating habits before she or he developed an eating disorder.

Prior to illness, the eating habits of individuals with eating disorders varied widely. Some have always been picky eaters, some have always been healthy eaters, others have been carefree eaters, and pretty commonly, your child, like most of us, loved to eat. In fact, for some, it is this love of eating that is scary for them: they may fear that their great love of food will make it difficult for them to stop eating once they have started. Through the course of treatment, your child will have some of these myths dispelled and will gain knowledge of what healthy eating really means. Because of this (more knowledge), **they won't go back to the way they ate before the illness. They can't go back to the totally "innocent" eating of youth.** However, nutrition knowledge, if used wisely, is a GOOD thing, not a bad thing. **There is nothing wrong with being a healthy eater. There are problems with being a FEARFUL EATER or a RIGID EATER.** We hope we will clarify the difference.

Fortunately or unfortunately, time always moves forward, and hopefully, we are learning things each step of the way. As your child's eating habits have changed as a result of this illness, we usually find two things have happened:

1. They have acquired more knowledge of nutrition.
2. They have distorted and exaggerated this nutrition knowledge so, while ill, this exaggerated knowledge is not used in a healthy manner.

Bottom line: accept the stage they are at NOW and move forward with them. It doesn't help your child to stay stuck in the past. Instead, the following steps are often used to improve the nutritional quality of someone with an eating disorder.

SUGGESTION BOX

Working as a Team During Meal Management: THE FOOD

♦   The first concern in restoring the health of someone with an eating disorder is the AMOUNT OF FOOD not the TYPE OF FOOD.

- It is fine if, in the beginning, your child continues to eat some safe foods **provided he or she is getting all the calories needed and there is regular progress toward increasing   the amount of food.**
- **However, be warned: safe foods don't have many calories. It is very hard to get everything with safe foods. The next chapter clarifies this.**

♦   As the meal planner, make balanced, healthy meals (a protein, a starch, a fruit and/or vegetable, and dairy); however, make sure your child can make a meal out of what is served given her/his stage on the "fear list."

- There is no right way to do this. However, usually a meal is composed of several items: some which may be more comfortable than others. Whether you prepare ONE item that is safer depends on the age of your child and the stage of the illness. Taking   baby steps is appropriate if the family is working as a team and your child is a member of that team. However, if the illness has been going on for a while, and your child's "membership" has been questionable (you feel you've been the hardest working member for a long time), then making something safe is NOT appropriate. Use your gut on this one. You know ☺.
- For example, consider a meal of grilled chicken, pasta and sauce, and vegetables. In the beginning your child may have the sauce as a fear food that is targeted as skills increase.

Middle/late adolescence (roughly 15-18 years)

Does our advice differ as your children get older? Yes and no. The basic strategies are the same, however, the older the child, the more input they have in terms of things they feel are helpful or unhelpful -with one very important caveat: we don't reinforce or follow your child's advice when that advice is given from the point of view of their illness. Before you get all worked up asking yourself "but how do you know...?" I'll tell you. You don't. You try listening to their advice in helping them through mealtimes and then you see what happens. Then, you tweak your approach based on what you observe. If listening to your child results in increased bargaining, conflict, and negotiation, you point that out and state that his/her opinion does not seem to be coming from a place of health so you need to step in a bit. Consider the example on the following page.

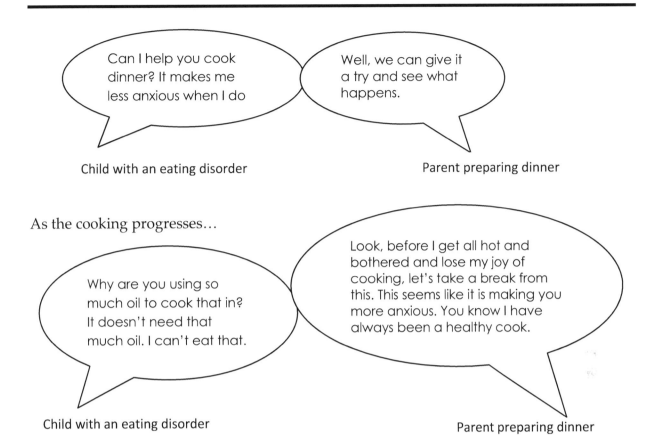

As the cooking progresses...

Your Child's Age and Meal Management

The basic formula is this: the older they are, the more their opinion is considered in the management of the illness. You implement their suggestions; see if they result in increased health.   If they do, you go with it; if they don't, you adapt and try something else (which often involves stepping in with greater support).

Trap #3: Mealtimes have become awful and I don't want to do them anymore!

As someone who was in charge of meal management on an inpatient unit of an eating disorder program for several years, all I can say is, I can relate. Not pleasant. However, there are some strategies that may be helpful. Here's another tip box to the rescue!! We actually devote a full chapter to healthy mealtimes; however, here are some quick tips to help you to avoid some pitfalls.

SUGGESTION BOX
Mealtime Coping Strategies During a Meal

DON'T talk about food or how much your child is eating during the meal. Why? Your child is already approaching something that causes him or her a lot of anxiety by joining the family for a meal and eating it. Talking about what is fearful when the individual is in a high state of arousal can make the fear stronger. Think DISTRACTION.

DON'T stare at your child's every move. Why? Would you want to be stared at while you eat? Enough said.

DON'T address how much your child has eaten (if that is your agreement) until after s/he has indicated s/he is finished. **HOW** and **WHY?** Talk about this BEFORE the meal and not right before. Plan what you will try in advance as during the meal your child is often too anxious to give good advice. Try it. See how it goes. Tweak it. Try again.

DO talk about anything else. **WHY?** Distraction at mealtimes is very helpful. There are so many things to talk about: what your children are studying in school, what is happening at your job, an event in the news, books you are reading, something you saw on television, information about fellow family members, sporting events, planning a family excursion, planning an "afternoon vacation" to give family members a break, a difficult situation at work that you could use advice with, the list goes on and on. Need more help? Order the UNGAME; it's a great conversation starter game!

DO role model healthy eating in accordance with YOUR appetite – not trying to match your child. **WHY?** Individuals with eating disorders often try to use events around them to regulate their behavior rather than turning inward and reading their own cues. Thus, they often calibrate how much they eat based on what others are eating around them – usually trying to eat the least. Don't play this game. Listen to your own body. Eat until YOU are full. If your child challenges you, explain this.

Trap #4: She or he cooks but doesn't eat.

Nope. You cook it, you have to try it. Period. Many the plate of cookies I have sent away when a patient will not join me in having one. Otherwise that supports the wrong message: we shouldn't put the needs of others ahead when our own health is failing. Generosity and giving come with health and balance.

Trap #5. My Child's Behaviors at Mealtimes Are Driving Me Insane.

To help your child, we need to understand a bit about the starvation process. Some eating behaviors (like cutting up your food into teeny, tiny pieces; talking about food all the time, collecting recipes) are an artifact of the starved state and will decrease when your child either gets to a healthy weight or loses the "restricter" mentality (more on this in the next trap). In addition, choose your battles. If you are addressing challenging issues, these behaviors may be annoying, but they should not be the focus. Stick to the important stuff and we'll address these in time. Now, if neither of those two scenarios apply, which two? It is important to keep in mind that having an eating disorder does not give someone permission to be rude at the table. However, many annoying behaviors are actually things your child may do to lower his or her anxiety. The best thing to do is to describe what you observe OUTSIDE OF THE MEAL and work together on a plan to address it. Emphasize teamwork: if you are willing to spend your time, he or she needs to put in theirs as well. Believe it or not, it will be a huge relief for your child to have limits set on their food rituals. THEY DRIVE THEM CRAZY TOO! When should you just let them have these rituals? Take one thing at a time.

Trap #6. My Child Thinks S/He is Binge Eating.

Many individuals with eating disorders exhibit symptoms of binge eating: periods of eating in which they feel "out of control" or unable to stop eating. Sometimes this may involve more food than would be expected given a specific situation, sometimes your children's rules for what they should or should not eat are so extreme that even a minor transgression makes them feel "out of control" even though they haven't eaten very much.

What is the parent's role when dealing with eating "too much" food? Parents often wonder, if their child is underweight, whether they should interfere. Of course, yes and no. If a child has been food restricted, then "overeating" at times, would be expected as it would for any starved person who finally had access to food. However, because this experience is so scary for your child, we want you to help your child focus on the BEHAVIORS around eating rather than the AMOUNT consumed. Don't forget: your child may be starving and thus may need to eat a great deal of food. However, we don't want her fears of overeating to get in the way of progress. Thus, to help your child relearn how to eat in a healthy way, do what you would do when they are younger:

1.   Eat while sitting down at the table. Your child learns to learn to read her or his body's cues. This happens best when there are set eating times rather than have eating occur all day long. Grazing often makes your child feel out of control. Try to have eating occur at the table.

2.   Pause between servings. Sometimes individuals with eating disorders, especially those individuals who make themselves throw up after meals, eating very rapidly during meals and lose contact with their body and end of feeling overfull. They then panic and try to "get rid of the food" by self-inducing vomiting. You can talk with your child about cuing her to slow down if you notice. The key: DISCUSS STRATEGIES IN ADVANCE, NOT IN THE HEAT OF THE MOMENT. In this way, your child can check in with her hunger and determine whether her body needs more food.

3.   Reassure your child that we all under or overeat sometimes. Life is about balance.

If your child regularly engages in episodes of overeating large amounts of food, talk about this to your child BEFORE a binge episode occurs. Together you can make a strategy to deal with it. I have seen parents do many things which include some or all of the following:

a) Keeping high risk foods out of the home for a period of time until their child felt more stable.

b) Having the child come to the parent when they felt the urge and the two of them go on a walk around the block.

c) Having the child leave immediately after a meal was completed and go watch television with the other parent.

d) Using urges as a signal to have a good talk with the parents about what might be stressful that they are resorting to symptoms.

e) And on and on and on… Remember, there is no right answer. You try. You observe what happens. You tweak. You learn. You try again!

Key Points

- There is no single correct way to achieve a so called "healthy" diet.
- While certain foods have a much better nutrient profile than others, a "healthy" diet may be inclusive of all foods.
- There are certain expectations (eating disordered or not) around acceptable mealtime behavior.
- The concepts of balance, moderation, variety and common sense are key to overcoming rigid food rules.
- It is initially more critical to work toward increasing total calories than to focus on variety and balance (although these are also important to implement at some point).
- It is normal for individuals with eating disorders to have concerns about weight repletion and eating more (i.e. fear of eating out of control, fear that weight gain will continue beyond a healthy level, etc.) and, as parents, we can have open discussion surrounding these concerns.
- The family must not change their menu to accommodate the individual with the eating disorder, but yet must assure that this individual has access to some foods which they will eat (i.e. provide a balanced meal consisting of all needed components, with inclusion of foods compatible with stage the eating disordered individual is in).
- Parents have access to many different strategies and approaches and you have the freedom to tweak these strategies in order to find the best solution for you.
- The process of eating disorder recovery may be slow.

Weekly Goals

Don't lose sight of your own joy of eating and of cooking. Think of the factors that you will need to bring back your joy of cooking (maybe attend a cooking class, clear the family out of the house while you cook and blasting some music) and create that experience for yourself. You are an important role model of the joy of eating.

Questions and Answers

Q: What if I struggle with disordered eating myself?

A: This is a very difficult situation and I am sorry you are having to struggle with both your own and your child's eating. Despite this, this is truly a golden opportunity to make healthy eating a part of your home for EVERYBODY FOR ALL TIME. It will be a very valuable opportunity for you to be open about your own struggles and to role model how you are going to address your own fears while your child works on hers. This is role modeling several invaluable things: your willingness to take responsibility for things you struggle with, your willingness to do things differently, and your courage in facing fears.

Q: What if I am not ready to address my own eating?

A: This is an extremely important issue that may, in fact, interfere with your child's recovery. As such, it is imperative that you speak to a mental health professional about your uncertainties, because asking your child to overcome her eating disorder while you engage in disordered eating behavior is extremely challenging and probably not possible. I strongly suggest you get the support you need to help you traverse your own journey towards health.

Wisdom of the Week: My Gift to Myself

If you need to, it may be a good idea to speak with a mental health counselor regarding your own struggles. We are generally pretty nice people.

Date:

Remember our key guidelines
It's a process! Try, tweak, grow and learn.
Self-parenting: a necessary prerequisite for other parenting.
Learn how to SURF The WAVE!
Remain genuine.

Unhealthy or unhelpful behavior I will discuss WITH my child this week and our plan to address it.

Eats too little	Eats too little variety	Exercises too much
Throws up after meals	Doesn't get enough sleep	Doesn't set limits
Abuses laxatives	Engages in self-harm	Other

Possible Suggestions of How to Address:

☐ Ignore it
☐ Have a discussion about needed change in behavior
   (discuss a future, necessary, logical consequence given the severity of the behavior)
☐ Implement a logical consequence (reminding your child of the importance of health before anything)
☐ Appeal to your child's inner wisdom (have a discussion with your child about what you have observed, why you are concerned, the change in behavior expected)
☐ Reverse Time-Out (you leave)
☐ Group Time-Out (everyone leaves for 10 minutes)
☐ Regrouping (family meeting to get out of power struggle)
☐ Humor

My Plan:

Would a discussion be a good idea?

Heathy Coping Strategy I will address with my child this week and my plan to address it.

Express negative emotions effectively	Ask for more help	Set more limits (cut down study time, set a regular bedtime, cut out an activity)
Express an opinion- even if someone may disagree	Be more considerate of others	Place more realistic demands on oneself (consider the cost, not whether the demands are achieved)
Get a better balance of work and leisure	View a situation with curiosity rather than with criticism	Manage disappointing results
Share a vulnerability with someone	Embrace and learn from mistakes rather than running from them	Resolve a conflict
Tune in and respond more to what your feelings are telling you	Take more pride in oneself (being a more respectful self-parent)	Strut
Be Silly or just take yourself less seriously	Smile at your reflection	Initiate plans
Try something new	Get Messy	Break a ritual
Get more sleep	Other	Other

Possible Suggestions:	**My Plan:**
☐ Positive attention when takes a step toward behavior ☐ One-on-one time outside of eating disorder stuff ☐ Earning a logical privilege given increased health ☐ Praise and STOP – no BUTS ☐ Role Model Behavior Yourself ☐ Open the door for a discussion ☐ Set a limit ☐ Offer to teach ☐ Other	

Heathy Coping Strategy I will Role Model this week.

Possible Suggestions:	**My Plan:**
☐ Delegate something. ☐ Say 'no' to some things. ☐ Be honest with my feelings. ☐ Express my feelings when not on the wave. ☐ Ask for help. ☐ Set healthy limits between my needs and those of others. ☐ Listen with full attention. ☐ Praise and STOP. ☐ Say "I'm sorry" with no excuses. ☐ Allow family members to make mistakes without jumping in. ☐ Be consistent. ☐ Address negative self-talk. ☐ Be reliable.	

Self-care Strategy I will implement this week

Possible Suggestions:	**My Plan:**
☐ Make regular mealtimes a priority. ☐ Set a regular bedtime. ☐ Learn a new hobby. ☐ Spend some time with my friends. ☐ Spend time ALONE with my spouse. ☐ Set a regular time I stop work each day. ☐ Take weekends off. ☐ Buy something for myself. ☐ Exercise in a MODERATE manner. ☐ Take pride in my physical appearance.	No lame excuses!!

TIP OF THE WEEK: Work to Keep the Sacredness of Mealtimes.

CHAPTER SIX: Understanding Behavior

Where You Are

- ✓ You have finished your first step. You have learned more about the program.

- ✓ You have learned more about the stages of parenting and how eating disorders take your child off the path of healthy growth.

- ✓ You have learned about strategies of parenting and emotion regulation that can help you be more effective in your role.

- ✓ You have learned about healthy nutrition and how this gets confused by your child's disorder.

Congratulations!!

You are getting very wise. Now we help you put it all together by giving you a better understanding of human behavior. When you better understand WHY people do the things they do, finding a solution is a lot easier.

Key Messages

Whenever you feel overwhelmed, take a step back and remember our main messages. They should help to direct you where you need to go.

It's a process: try, tweak, learn, grow.
Self-parenting: a necessary step for other-parenting.
Stay off the wave.
Stay genuine.

Topic: Behavior Management

Behavior management? Why in the world are we talking about something that you have been doing for years with your children? Well, eating disorders and the children most likely to develop an eating disorder pose some interesting challenges for parents. First, the behaviors that are part of an eating disorder (refusing to eat, throwing up after meals, etc.) SEEM more confusing to manage than behaviors like staying out past curfew, swearing to your parent, etc. Second, often (but not always), children who develop eating disorders have always been the "good kids." You may have never HAD to use behavioral management strategies because these children always did what they were supposed to do! Third, individuals who develop eating disorders often do something puzzling: they do TOO MUCH of a GOOD THING. As I hope you are learning, too much of ANYTHING is a problem. Thus, we need to set limits on too much of a good thing as much as we need to set limits on A LITTLE of an UNHEALTHY thing. Learning to manage an eating disorder is about learning to decrease unhealthy behavior and increase healthy behavior. As you probably have noticed by now, this is what we seek to do with all behavior. Our aim with ourselves, our children, our significant others ... is to decrease behaviors that are harmful or not helpful and to replace those behaviors with helpful behaviors. This chapter will teach you general strategies of behavior management so that you will be confident in applying the knowledge you have learned to new situations that arise. As you will see, whenever you encounter a problem, you can go through the following steps and begin to determine how to approach the problem and solve it. Odds are you already know all of this. If so, many parents just find their child's disorder has thrown them "off balance" a little and they just need a friendly reminder to get back on track. Perhaps we'll also have some useful tips you have not thought of before....

Part I: Addressing Unhealthy Behaviors

Keep Your Eye on the Ball

Our primary goal in helping your child with an eating disorder is restoring physical and mental health. Because of the seriousness of these illnesses on physical health, we need to make sure to maintain our focus on helping your child to restore healthy nutrition. Our IMMEDIATE goal is for your child to eat healthy meals and snacks, to eat enough food to maintain health, and exercise moderately. Thus, our primary mission is to help your child have an adequate breakfast, lunch, dinner and snacks. Anything that gets in the way of this happening gets eliminated or rescheduled. Thus, when you find yourself getting all confused and trying to fit medical appointments around school, extracurricular activities, etc., you need to step back and say "Wait a minute. If my child is not healthy, nothing else matters. Let's deal with health. The rest will work itself out in due time."

TIP BOX

There are many ways to skin a cat.

Parents often get very concerned about minimizing the impact of their child's illness on the rest of their lives. From experience, I can tell you that these things are not true. First of all, the majority of people go through hard times. Going through a hard time does not mean the rest of your life is destroyed. In fact, it could mean just the opposite as the growth that occurs during the "rough period" often makes an individual so much stronger to deal with what life has to offer. However, if a family does not invest their energy in working on the problems, and, instead, focuses continually on the future, ironically, that may lengthen the rough period and decrease the amount of learning that occurs.

Logical Consequences

As your family makes a plan to increase the health of your child, keep in mind that this is not a power struggle. Instead, it is you working with your child as a team to beat this disorder. However, if your child is not ready to be a team player, then the plans to improve health need to be made without the benefit of his or her input. In such cases, there may be a need to use logical consequences. Logical consequences are just what they sound like: they are the consequences that naturally follow when certain things happen. The chart on the following page gives you an example of some eating disorder behaviors and the logical consequences that may naturally follow. Keep in mind, the family decided on these together unless the child wasn't willing to contribute and then the parents decided on their own.

Eating Disorder Behavior	Logical Consequence	Why is this Logical?
Person is not able to eat enough food at a meal.	He goes up to bed and rests to regain his strength so he has enough energy to battle the disorder at the next meal.	Someone who is not able to eat is very, very sick. A person like that in a hospital would often be on feeding tube or some severe measure to restore health. Thus, it does not make sense for someone who cannot eat properly to be doing the other things a healthy person does because this person is not healthy.
Person throws up after meals.	Parents stay with their child for 90 minutes after meals to provide extra support.	This child is struggling with her illness following meals and needs added support. The parents jump in and provide it.
Person is not able to eat meals when away from home.	This child is required to eat meals at home.	This one is pretty easy to reason through. ☺
Person is not able to exercise a moderate amount.	Exercise is not permitted until the child feels comfortable turning his behavior on and off. When he starts to exercise again, a parent or support person goes with.	Individuals with eating disorders struggle with their "on" and "off" button. Often first things need to be removed until a better "switch" can be taught.
Person wants to exchange a higher calorie item for a lower calorie item	Parents give the child 2 or 3 food exchange items of equal calories.	Parents don't negotiate with an eating disorder. Trying to swap for lower calories is definitely a sign your child is on the top of the eating disorder wave.
Person is not gaining weight although underweight and was continuing to participate in dance class.	Dance lessons are not permitted until weight is restored to healthy limits.	A person too sick to eat is too sick to dance. Health comes before dance.

Hopefully this is starting to make sense.

Barriers to Extinction

Just like an animal who becomes extinct, a behavior becomes extinct (no longer exists) when that behavior stops being associated with things we want or with ending things we didn't want. In order for this process to happen, there are three essential ingredients: consistency, immediacy, and specificity. Let's take a look at each.

Consistency: The behavior should ALWAYS be followed by the consequence. "Every time my child throws up after her meal, she will go lie down to restore her strength for the next meal or until she has the strength to drink some nutritional supplement to replace her lost nourishment." "Every time Nancy says a curse word, she gets sent to her room." (Actually, it used to be the 'mouth washed out with soap' routine).

Immediacy: The behavior should be followed by the logical consequence as closely as possible to when the behavior occurred. This makes it easier for your child as he or she experiences the immediate impact of his/her behavior. "Every time my child speaks to me in a rude tone, I immediately end the conversation and request to resume it later when she can be polite."

Specificity: The eating disorder needs to know the rules. Vague rules end up in a million "eating disorder excuses" that leave you backed into a corner. Specific rules leave no room for negotiation. "If you throw up after a meal, it shows your strength is compromised, so we have two options: to rest until you are ready to be nourished or to replace what your body just lost with a substitute."

Summary of Part I

This first section outlined setting up an immediate plan to address your child's symptoms. This next section focuses on helping you to understand how your child's symptoms help her cope so you and your child can develop a more long-range strategy to both manage the symptom and practice healthier coping. Enjoy!

Part II: Understanding Unhealthy Behaviors and Developing Coping Strategies

In an earlier section, we introduced you to the general laws of behavior. It is helpful to keep these in mind as we try to better understand your child's illness.

Notice General Patterns

When you are trying to learn more about your child's eating disorder behaviors, your first task is to learn when the toughest times are for your child. Does he struggle more at night than in the morning? More at lunch? More at breakfast? How do you find out? Ask your child! Explore this together. He knows.

Here are some things I have heard individuals with eating disorders say:

> "Breakfasts are easy because I am hungry for it and the foods are pretty safe."

> "I have a tough time with eating early in the day because I am afraid that if I eat too much, then I'll have nothing left for the evening and then end up overeating. I save my calories and try to eat most of it at the end of the day."

> "All meals suck."

What do you do when you have learned something about your child's patterns? Well, we call times when your child's symptoms get worse "high risk situations." To minimize the likelihood of your child struggling during these times, you make a plan! The plan should focus on increasing support or thinking through strategies **in advance** regarding tough periods. Some options to plan for high risk periods in advance may include:

- Increasing your attendance at these times
- Planning activities to do together when the meal is over (this is particularly helpful if your child struggles with vomiting after meals)
- Leaving the house to go on a drive
- Planning meals in advance
- Removing high risk food items from the house

The goal is to make this a discussion with your child. However, if your child is not willing or not ready to be a part of that discussion, then you will just need to inform her that you will have to make the choice without the benefit of her input because a plan needs to be made. Her health is too compromised to do anything less.

Tip Box Individuals with eating disorders struggle a great deal with offering input into any type of plan. This is because their disorder "pressures them" into making the choice that is the "most disordered" while the healthy part of them struggles to please you. Thus, they often just feel stuck. Your best strategy is to give your child a multiple choice option: they have to choose from the choices you offer them, but at least the range of options is now A LOT easier.

Here is an example. Parent is on the left. In this situation, the family finds out that their child's weight was down from last week.

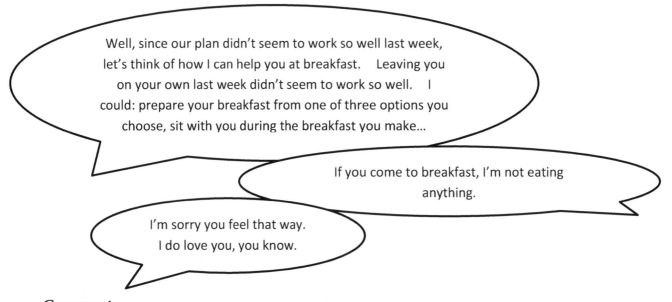

Well, since our plan didn't seem to work so well last week, let's think of how I can help you at breakfast. Leaving you on your own last week didn't seem to work so well. I could: prepare your breakfast from one of three options you choose, sit with you during the breakfast you make...

If you come to breakfast, I'm not eating anything.

I'm sorry you feel that way. I do love you, you know.

Comments

Of course, the parent will show up at breakfast tomorrow despite the child's protests. Why? Well, there was no use in a logical discussion at that point as the child was clearly on the wave. Another thing this parent did that works well: he made everything a "we" to remind his child this is a family problem, not just the child's problem.

The take home message from this discussion is to first learn about **general patterns** of difficulty (e.g. times of day, times of week) of your child's disorder. If so, we need to make special plans for these times. This helps us with GENERAL management. A more complicated issue is learning about how your child's symptoms help him or her to cope with the stresses of life.

> **TIP BOX**
> Behavior therapists refer to situations that make a behavior MORE or LESS likely to occur as "antecedents". Learning about these factors is important as these factors give us clues about why the behavior is occurring and how to manage it. Knowledge about antecedents can help us to outsmart unhealthy behavior BEFORE it happens. We all do this already without realizing it. For example, whenever I have to meet with the chairman of my department (often stressful), I always plan to go shoe shopping (or browsing) later in the day. Pairing something delightful with something dreaded can take away a lot of the distress!

Notice Fluctuating Patterns

Remember the Eating Disorder Wave? When we discussed the wave for your child, we mentioned how upsetting events may send your child up the wave and make her more sensitive to eating disorder "cues." It is the events that ORIGINALLY upset your child that we need to learn more about. If we can teach your child to cope more effectively with the things in her daily experiences that upset her, then she won't need her eating disorder to cope, right? Sounds easy, but your child is not sensitive to changes in her emotions. However, she IS VERY sensitive to the volume of her eating disorder at any given moment. We use EATING DISORDER volume as a RED FLAG that something is bothering her. We just need to work as a team to figure it out.

All of us are sometimes upset and we just don't know why. If we **are** able to figure it out, often we get stuck about what to do about it. We'll tackle both of these issues. By the end of this chapter, you'll be able to solve all your problems (exaggeration for dramatic effect).

> **TIP BOX**
> There are two parts to feeling confident about our ability to handle life's challenges: we have to be in touch with ourselves to figure out what's wrong and we have to know what to do about it! The trick: you have to go back and retrace your steps to figure out what made you climb the wave in the first place!

When? Well, it might go something like this. Let's say your child has had a relatively easy time managing things over the past few days, but today has really been a struggle.

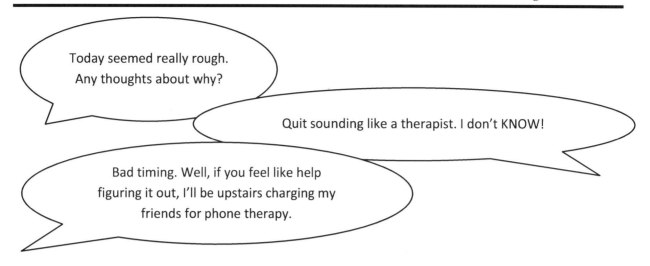

So, after repeating this scenario on several occasions, your child finally takes you up on your offer. What to do?

Well, we haven't finished our discussion of the wave, yet. We really have not explained one of the most important parts of the Wave (I don't know if you always want this in caps): once you come down from the wave without injury, you need to go back and figure out what bothered you in the first place. Your job is then to make a plan to address the situation.

WHY??? Our emotions give us a message about ourselves and communicate a need we have. They are a signal that something is going on. In order for us to benefit from the message of our emotions, learn more about ourselves, and develop a sense of self-trust, we have to listen to this message and respond to it. Then the message is delivered and the emotion will end, or decrease. As it sounds, this involves calmness, patience, and thoughtfulness, not a top of the wave task to be sure! So, our first job is to get off the wave. Then, we can investigate what this emotion is trying to tell us.

Although this seems horribly complicated, we can actually take a very logical process to do this. Well, you have to play detective.

I usually instruct the people I work with to do a "chain analysis" to figure out at one point their mood shifted – either from good to bad or from bad to worse. A chain analysis is a play-by-play analysis of your day. Your goal is to figure out what was upsetting you by isolating the period of the day when your mood shifted. We will walk you through a sample chain analysis.

It usually goes something like this:

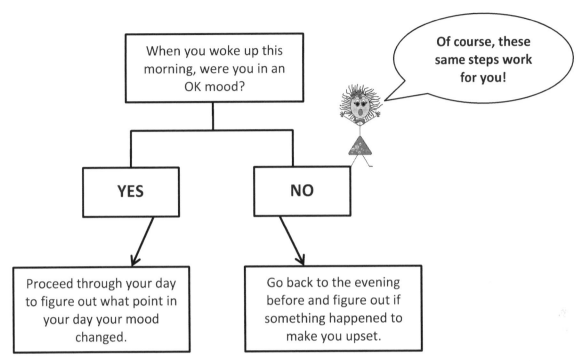

...and so on and so. Your goal is to pinpoint the time of day your mood changed from good to bad, from bad to worse, etc.

Next, you have to figure out what happened. Basically, there are three things that could have happened:

1. You have a problem with something about yourself.
2. You have a problem with someone else.
3. You have a problem with the environment.

We go through a detailed analysis of strategies of each of these situations in Chapters 15 and 16, when we become a professional surfer. For now, we're keeping it simple. Here's an example of this in action, then we'll summarize the steps.

An Example

You notice your child is having a particularly difficult day. You focus on meal management strategies as usual (your plan is to be present during meals and to spend time together following meals to help him to avoid vomiting). However, your child is doing more protesting than usual and seems more agitated than usual. AFTER THE MEAL IS OVER, and after your child seems more settled, you open the door for a discussion about why the day was hard. If your child feels like discussing it, you play detective, help him think through what was wrong, and help him make a plan to address it. If he is not ready to talk, you express your willingness to talk whenever he feels like it AND YOU DROP IT FOR NOW. (When it comes to talking, timing is KEY. You can't make someone talk when they don't feel like it and when parents try to push it, it is ANNOYING.). When he is ready, you decide on a plan. Your child tries it. You talk about how it went and keep the parts that worked and tweak the parts that didn't work!

The Steps of Problem Solving, Wave Style

1. You notice your child is having a particularly tough time.
2. You make sure you are particularly consistent regarding meal management strategies (and may even increase the level of support).
3. After the meal is completed and your child seems at a point where he can be logical, you present your observations and offer to help figure out the problem.
4. When your child is ready, you play detective together and figure out the point in the day (or the evening before), when your child's mood shifted from good to bad or from bad to worse.
5. You identify the event, person, or thought that caused the mood shift and you brainstorm a plan to address the situation.
6. Your child tries the plan.
7. You talk about how it went, you keep the part that works and revise the part that didn't.
8. You try again.
9. You role model this with circumstances in your own life that are upsetting.

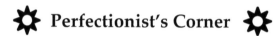 **Perfectionist's Corner**

Perfectionist: What if my child and I make the wrong decision?

Voice of Reason: There actually is no "right" decision. You learn from doing. You pick SOMETHING. You try it. You learn from the experience and tweak your approach. It may not turn out as well as you would have hoped the first time. But you couldn't possibly know that in advance, could you? You have to take the risk of trying to learn anything.

Perfectionist: This makes a lot of sense. However, my child and I are exhausted. When she has finally calmed down, I don't want to bring things up that are upsetting. I want to let her enjoy the moment.

Voice of Reason: I don't blame you one bit and, in your shoes, I would feel the same. However, there is a difference between "short term pain" and "long term gain." In order for your child to develop healthy coping strategies, we have to have the courage to look at what bothered us and work through it, even if thinking about it increases our distress temporarily. If we don't do that, the problem just simmers below the surface, negatively impacting our health and our relationships and just waiting for an opportunity to erupt into a full blown tidal wave!

When? Timing, timing, timing...

We have made reference to the importance of timing, but we just want to make sure we make that point clear. You can't force someone to talk. People have different surfing abilities. Some people can go through a tidal wave and immediately want to discuss what happened. Some people need to let the experience simmer for a few days and then go back and revisit it. Neither strategy is right nor wrong, so long as you go back and look at the issue at some point. When you and someone you love have different strategies, you have to respect each others limits and sometimes, WAIT.

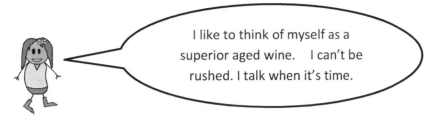

I like to think of myself as a superior aged wine.   I can't be rushed. I talk when it's time.

Before we leave, let's look at a sample homework sheet. Perhaps the logic of these strategies is starting to make more sense now. Here's a sample.

Unhealthy behavior I will address in my child: **not eating enough food.**	
☒ Have a discussion about the plan. ☐ Ignore it.	Plan: I will have a talk with my child about the need for us the follow the doctor's recommendations regarding her meal plan, as for her input about whether she would like it done in large meals or smaller meals and frequent snacks and will remind her about the importance of health above all when she tries to negotiate fewer calories. If she is unable to do this I will keep her home from school that day to rest and regain her strength.
Healthy behavior I will address in my child	
☒ Difficulty asking for help.	Plan: I will offer my child ways I can be helpful with meal times using a multiple choice strategy that she can pick fro as she may have difficulties thinking of ways I can help on her own.
Healthy behavior I will role model.	
☒ Difficulty asking for help	Plan: I will ask my friends for help with car pools this week and will refuse to do some volunteering at the school due to limited time.
Nice thing I will do for myself this week.	
☒ Stake out my own territory.	Plan: I will pick a spot in my home (finally) to designate as my own spot and no one is to bother me when I am there. I'll buy a few things to decorate it.

Key Points

Hopefully, these rules make a lot more sense now.

1. When there is a behavior that you are trying to end or decrease, you first have to play detective and figure out what the person gets out of performing the behavior.
2. Then, when your child is ready, make a plan to address the situation that caused the problem in the first place.
3. Timing is important.
4. REINFORCE HEALTHY BEHAVIOR, EXTINGUISH UNHEALTHY BEHAVIOR!

Weekly Goals

1. Think about the eating disorder symptoms you are targeting. Think about some skills your child needs to develop (asking for help or support, setting limits on self, etc.). Make some goals **for your child (the greater your child's level of motivation and participation, the more you involve them in goal setting with you. In the beginning, you will be doing more of the planning.)**
2. Think about some things **you** can role model in this section. Make some goals **for yourself.**
3. Think about your team. Decide who can help you with implementing these strategies and talk with them.
4. Then, talk to your child about your goals and how you will help. This is your planning meeting. Thus, before you go on, take some time to think through steps one and two. Then, head for the chair.
5. Use these goals to create your homework sheet on the following pages.

Questions and Answers

Q: I tried a plan and it didn't work. What do I do now? Guess your program doesn't work for my family, huh??

A: Of course it didn't work! Things never go as "perfectly" as we would like, do they? Remember one of our key mottos: It's a process! Your mission is to think through what you did, how it went, and to take away that 'all or nothing' thinking. Think about the parts of your plan that did not work. Think of any baby steps you took towards your goal. Think about the part of your plan that helped you to take those baby steps. Keep those. Tweak the rest. Make this a discussion, if you can.

Q: My child and I seem to be in a huge power struggle. She has lost all her privileges and doesn't seem to care. Now what do I do?

A: Yuck! What a terrible feeling. It seems like you and your child have gotten away from the whole "teamwork" mentality – something that is quite easy to do with these disorders. I would recommend the following steps:

Regrouping meeting with your child where you:

    i.   Emphasize your love and concern for your child's health.

   ii.   Take ownership of the mistakes you made and things you could have done differently.

  iii.   Resolve for everyone to start over from this point forward.

   iv.   Emphasis on the severity of this illness and your resolve not to let anything harm your child.

Wisdom of the Week: My Gift to Myself

Take out your social support inventory and reach out and touch somebody you haven't spoken to in awhile. An email, a call, a card – whatever works!!

GOALS FOR WEEK #6

Date:

Remember our key guidelines

It's a process! Try, tweak, grow and learn.

Self-parenting: a necessary prerequisite for other parenting.

Learn how to SURF The WAVE!

Remain genuine.

Unhealthy or unhelpful behavior I will discuss WITH my child this week and our plan to address it.

Eats too little	Eats too little variety	Exercises too much
Throws up after meals	Doesn't get enough sleep	Doesn't set limits
Abuses laxatives	Engages in self-harm	Other

Possible Suggestions of How to Address:

☐ Ignore it

☐ Have a discussion about needed change in behavior *(discuss a future, necessary, logical consequence given the severity of the behavior)*

☐ Implement a logical consequence (reminding your child of the importance of health before anything)

☐ Appeal to your child's inner wisdom (have a discussion with your child about what you have observed, why you are concerned, the change in behavior expected)

☐ Reverse Time-Out (you leave)

☐ Group Time-Out (everyone leaves for 10 minutes)

☐ Regrouping (family meeting to get out of power struggle)

☐ Humor

My Plan:

Would a discussion be a good idea?

Heathy Coping Strategy I will address with my child this week and my plan to address it.

Express negative emotions effectively	Ask for more help	Set more limits (cut down study time, set a regular bedtime, cut out an activity)
Express an opinion- even if someone may disagree	Be more considerate of others	Place more realistic demands on oneself (consider the cost, not whether the demands are achieved)
Get a better balance of work and leisure	View a situation with curiosity rather than with criticism	Manage disappointing results
Share a vulnerability with someone	Embrace and learn from mistakes rather than running from them	Resolve a conflict
Tune in and respond more to what your feelings are telling you	Take more pride in oneself (being a more respectful self-parent)	Strut
Be Silly or just take yourself less seriously	Smile at your reflection	Initiate plans
Try something new	Get Messy	Break a ritual
Get more sleep	Other	Other

Possible Suggestions:	**My Plan:**
☐ Positive attention when takes a step toward behavior ☐ One-on-one time outside of eating disorder stuff ☐ Earning a logical privilege given increased health ☐ Praise and STOP – no BUTS ☐ Role Model Behavior Yourself ☐ Open the door for a discussion ☐ Set a limit ☐ Offer to teach ☐ Other	

Heathy Coping Strategy I will Role Model this week.

Possible Suggestions:	**My Plan:**
☐ Delegate something. ☐ Say 'no' to some things. ☐ Be honest with my feelings. ☐ Express my feelings when not on the wave. ☐ Ask for help. ☐ Set healthy limits between my needs and those of others. ☐ Listen with full attention. ☐ Praise and STOP. ☐ Say "I'm sorry" with no excuses. ☐ Allow family members to make mistakes without jumping in. ☐ Be consistent. ☐ Address negative self-talk. ☐ Be reliable.	

Self-care Strategy I will implement this week

Possible Suggestions:	**My Plan:**
☐ Make regular mealtimes a priority. ☐ Set a regular bedtime. ☐ Learn a new hobby. ☐ Spend some time with my friends. ☐ Spend time ALONE with my spouse. ☐ Set a regular time I stop work each day. ☐ Take weekends off. ☐ Buy something for myself. ☐ Exercise in a MODERATE manner. ☐ Take pride in my physical appearance.	No lame excuses!!

TIP OF THE WEEK: Symptoms are signs there is a problem that needs solving.

CHAPTER SEVEN: Barriers to Behavior Change

Where You Are

- ✓ You have finished your first step. You have learned more about the program.
- ✓ You have learned more about the stages of parenting and how eating disorders take your child off the path of healthy growth.
- ✓ You have learned about strategies of parenting and emotion regulation that can help you be more effective in your role.
- ✓ You have learned about healthy nutrition and how this gets confused by your child's disorder.
- ✓ You have learned about behavior and he factors that keep it going.

Congratulations!!

You have really learned a ton so far.

Topic: Barriers to Behavior Change

The last chapter introduced you to behaviors that are helpful in managing this illness in the short term and understanding this illness in the longer term. This section focuses on some common patterns that get in the way of the families' ability to implement the most well-articulated of plans.

Barrier #1: Intermittent Reinforcement

The first factor we will discuss is called "**intermittent reinforcement.**" This occurs when we are INCONSISTENT in regard to the plan we designed to cope with unhealthy behavior. Sometimes we keep to the plan. Sometimes we don't. Think about this example:

You like to gamble. You play the slot machines. Most of the time (in fact the vast majority of the time), you lose money. You win every once in a while. Or, equally important, you see someone else win.

> **TIP BOX**
>
> **Being reinforce every once in a while is the greatest way to assure that a behavior will take a long time to go away. The individual thinks (or knows) that, sooner or later, they will get the reward if they just keep performing the behavior.**

The eating disorder **loves it** when you are inconsistent as the eating disorder is a gambler by nature. If the eating disorder thinks it can get away with something some of the time, then BY GOLLY! IT SURE IS GOING TO TRY ALL THE TIME. :)!!

Tee, hee. Dad has been losing his cool more often. It's only a matter of time before he gives up and then the house is mine!!!

Now, don't worry. Consistency is difficult. If you find you have been inconsistent about a rule, all is not lost. You just acknowledge to your child that you had trouble with the plan, you figure out what happened and you make a revised plan. This is actually a great opportunity to demonstrate to your child that mistakes are a valuable part of learning.

> **TIP BOX**
>
> **When you get frustrated, pull out a baby picture! It can help to bring out happy, fund memories and to share these with your child! It puts things in perspective.**

Barrier #2: Extinction Burst

Another **BARRIER** that can interfere with extinction unless you know about it is "EXTINCTION BURST." When one is trying to change a behavior, <u>initially you may see an increase in the behavior!!!</u>

If you think about this, this makes perfect sense. Before the rules changed, the unhelpful behavior resulted in a positive consequence. If that positive consequence does not occur, before an individual just gives up the behavior he might first try to **STRENGTHEN** the behavior to see if that works. A great example of this is if you have ever been speaking sternly with your child to try to get their attention. First you scream at them before you shift to a different strategy. Think about the temper tantrum example. If you initially ignore the tantrum (whereas you previously had given in), the tantrum is going to get LOUDER before it starts going away. We call this EXTINCTION BURST.

Unfortunately, many parents get nervous by this increase because they think that this is a sign that the new strategies are not working. Just be patient and consistent. You'll see. I have developed the "THREE DAY RULE" with the families I work with. It seems they are often tested for three days of extreme intensity before things settle down.

What Extinction Burst May *Look Like to You*	What Extinction Burst May *Feel Like for Your Child*
• **Increased arguing or negotiating around meals** • **Increased food rituals** • **Increased food refusals** • **More urges to throw up or exercise** • **Increased negative body image talk or "I feel fat" talk** • **You know the drill…..**	• **It may seem that the volume of the eating disorder in her head is getting louder and more critical** • **Increased sensations of bloating or fullness** • **Increased feelings of fatness** • **Increased anxiety or agitation**

It may be a good idea to warn your child about extinction burst. Then, she won't be nervous if the eating disorder initially gets louder before it starts to quiet down.

Tip Box: Reasonable Expectations

In some cases, your child may not have the skills to perform a healthy alternative behavior. In this case, you need to teach her those skills so she can replace the unhealthy behavior. Think about expressing negative emotions. If your child has never been good at expressing negative emotions, and then starts to express them, she might not express them very well. In fact, she may be downright rude. Our mission is to validate the feelings (she certainly has a right to be angry), and also to ask her to be more courteous with how she expresses it the next time she feels angry). Worry not! We get better at skills the more we practice.

Barrier #3 The Honeymoon Period

Ah yes. The honeymoon period. This is a time when all things seem to be going "perfectly." You set some new rules regarding what you expect in terms of behavior change. Your child happily follows along without so much as a peep of protest. Sound too good to be true? Well, it COULD be. Why??? There are a few reasons.

1. Your child (or the eating disorder) doesn't think you'll keep it up.
Your child knows patterns of past behavior. In addition, the eating disorder can be sneaky. He/she knows that maybe in the past, like the majority of parents, you have made a rule and not followed up with it. He/she also knows that you are human and get tired over time. How is this related to the honeymoon period? Well, your child may go "along with things" in the beginning, figuring that you will get comfortable and let your guard down, or as most of us do, just get tired and not enforce the rules you have set.

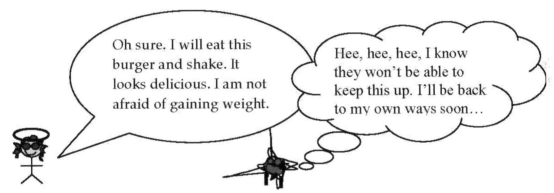

So what's the solution? Just be aware. Things that are difficult are worth fighting for, and the fight may be drawn out sometimes. Eating disorders are scary. When your child starts eating again, you so want to believe the crisis is over that you may back off too quickly. You can avoid any problems with this by following the simple formula: a reminder about the "Dance of Parenting." We haven't talked about the dance in several chapters, so let's revisit it for a moment.

The simple dance of parenting: When to Lean In, When to Step Back

There are no right answers to this. This is a trial and error process. You give your child a trial with a new freedom. If she demonstrates she can handle it, she gets to keep the freedom. If she demonstrates that it is too much right now, you take a step back and assist until she and you are ready to try again.

The "more elaborate" dance of parenting

More specifically, the way anyone gains a new freedom is he demonstrates he has the skills to handle it.
1. First you teach him the new skill.
2. You practice the new skill with him.
3. You step back and let him try the new skill on his own.

4. When you do this, one of three things may happen.
    a. He shows that not only can he perform the skill this time, but he can perform the skill over time. Result: You allow your child to continue to perform the activity and over time, increase his level of responsibility.
    b. She shows she can perform the skill in the short term, but she has difficulty maintaining the skill over time. Result: Praise their initial effort, point out where performance has fallen off, give her a chance to improve and if she doesn't bounce back, you have to take back the responsibility for that skill for a while until it is time to try again.
    c. He is just not ready yet and you lean in for a bit longer.

Barrier #4: Lack of Teamwork

The fourth barrier that we often see is a lack of teamwork. This lack of teamwork can occur between the parents and their child with the eating disorder, between the parents and their children without the disorder, or between the parents themselves. Let's think about what teamwork is, what it takes, and what to do in each of these cases.

Teamwork happens when people work together to achieve a common goal. Sounds simple enough, eh? If only. For teamwork to happen, it takes several things.

1. **The team members agree on the goal.**

This seems obvious, but oftentimes people don't work as a team because they don't realize they are working for different things. The only way to know this is to talk about it. Do both of you agree on the most effective way to bring your family back to health? Do you have different beliefs? This is expected and OK so long as you talk about it and work on a compromise.

<u>**Goal: Define Your Goals.**</u>

2. **The team members discuss disagreements about the goal and the plan.**
Working as a team takes practice. You start with one plan. It doesn't work. You try another. A good team shares responsibility when things don't go well. They DON'T blame each other. They don't keep their opinions to themselves. Instead, they discuss what happened, respect the other members, and tweak the plan.

<u>**Goal: Share successes and missteps and talk about them.**</u>

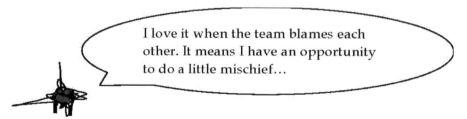

I love it when the team blames each other. It means I have an opportunity to do a little mischief…

3. **The team members are open to feedback from the other team members.**
In order for a team to be able to give each other feedback, the members have to be

willing to TAKE feedback. This means you are open to learning. Hopefully, we are making good progress on this! Once you REALLY BELIEVE this is all a part of a learning process, everything gets A LOT easier.

Goal: <u>**Be open-minded.**</u>

4. **Team members listen to each other and give feedback respectfully.**

Nobody has all the answers. Nobody knows what someone else is thinking. Each team member may have a valuable idea to contribute. We have to be willing to really hear what each team member has to say and to consider where he or she is coming from. If we do this, that team member will be more willing to listen to our idea.

Goal: <u>**Listen for understanding.**</u>

5. **Team members are willing to tweak the plan.**

See above. Things get better over time. Be prepared to take baby steps.

Goal: <u>**Patience.**</u>

So let's say the father thinks the mother should be making more high calories meals for dinner for their child with an eating disorder. Rather than say anything, he makes insulting comments to the mom about babying their daughter. Teamwork? No way. What would be more helpful? Well, away from their daughter, the father could discuss his confusion about the menu and ask about making higher calorie dinners. The mom listens. She considers his opinion. She gives her opinion. They reach a common understanding and then discuss the plan with their child. Sound ideal? You bet! Can you do it? You bet.

You go through these same steps when it feels like any of your children is not acting like a part of the team. Discuss, listen, express your side; tweak and try again.

Tip Box

As we have mentioned, teamwork involves listening and considering everyone's opinion. However, considering someone else's opinion means you understand their position. However, if their position is one that advocates unhealthy things, then we don't enter their opinion into the plan. We <u>**never**</u> compromise on health.

Pulling It All Together

Are you feeling overwhelmed by the amount of skills you have learned? Worry not! Don't forget our key principles. All we have taught you goes back to these four things. If you master these, you are SET!

Key Messages

It's a process: try, tweak, learn, grow.
Self-parenting: a necessary step for other-parenting.
Stay off the wave.
Stay genuine.

Key Points

1. An Off the C.U.F.F. approach is a great style to practice in managing your child's eating disorder.
2. This is a family mission: the whole family bonding together to battle this disorder.
3. Discuss strategies and seek your child's input AS LONG AS that input comes from a place of health and not illness. There is no negotiation with an eating disorder, but your child can give healthy input.
4. Consider your child's age in the degree of input, but don't miscommunicate your values. Health comes first.
5. Whenever the plan is unclear, it's time to regroup and re-plan (otherwise known as a "family discussion, a family car ride, a letter to your child – do what works).
6. Your child is not his or her disorder – no matter what s/he feels in the moment. When the eating disorder is loud, that is a moment of extreme emotional intensity for your child and they may not have clarity.

Weekly Goals

When you feel your family is not acting as a team, take a step back, consider the steps and figure out where the teamwork is beginning to fall apart.

Questions and Answers

Q: What if my spouse and I have very different opinions regarding how to get our child healthy and there doesn't seem to be room for compromise?

A: Ah, the answer to that dilemma is actually an EXPERIENCE as we never know what will work until we try it out! So, you decide that you will consistently try your way or your spouse's way for a period of time and you see what happens. If that strategy is bringing your child closer towards health, stick with it. If not, tweak it, which may involve incorporating your plan.

"Bonus Tip"

Parents sometimes get very nervous then they feel that the eating disorder is gaining some ground. Maybe everybody was tired and had a bad week, maybe the moon was full, maybe ....not to worry!! You can always recoup your losses. You can announce that you are aware that it was a bad week and that everybody is starting fresh with the next meal, and move on or you can just think this in your head. We all could use fresh starts now and again! A similar strategy, what I call "A GROUP TIME OUT" is one of the more effective ways to manage a situation in which everyone is riding the emotional wave. An example is below.

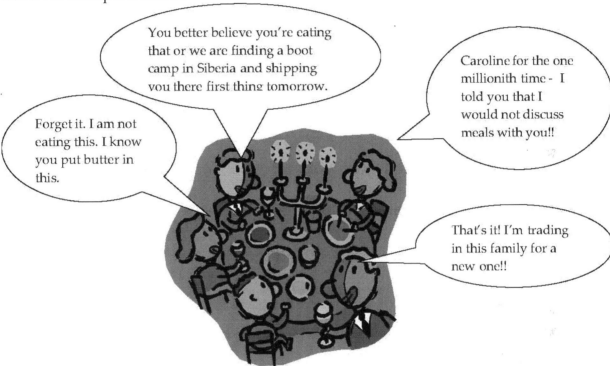

In this strategy, the point is that everyone needs to take a time-out to calm down and clear their head so the meal can start over. Usually the best way to do this is for everyone to leave the table for 10 minutes, go to their respective corners (rooms), do whatever works to calm down and then return. The hardest part is that someone has to be **mature enough** to call the group time-out.

Date:

Remember our key guidelines
It's a process! Try, tweak, grow and learn.
Self-parenting: a necessary prerequisite for other parenting.
Learn how to SURF The WAVE!
Remain genuine.

Unhealthy or unhelpful behavior I will discuss WITH my child this week and our plan to address it.

Eats too little	Eats too little variety	Exercises too much
Throws up after meals	Doesn't get enough sleep	Doesn't set limits
Abuses laxatives	Engages in self-harm	Other

Possible Suggestions of How to Address:

☐ Ignore it
☐ Have a discussion about needed change in behavior
(discuss a future, necessary, logical consequence given the severity of the behavior)
☐ Implement a logical consequence (reminding your child of the importance of health before anything)
☐ Appeal to your child's inner wisdom (have a discussion with your child about what you have observed, why you are concerned, the change in behavior expected)
☐ Reverse Time-Out (you leave)
☐ Group Time-Out (everyone leaves for 10 minutes)
☐ Regrouping (family meeting to get out of power struggle)
☐ Humor

My Plan:

Would a discussion be a good idea?

Heathy Coping Strategy I will address with my child this week and my plan to address it.

Express negative emotions effectively	Ask for more help	Set more limits (cut down study time, set a regular bedtime, cut out an activity)
Express an opinion- even if someone may disagree	Be more considerate of others	Place more realistic demands on oneself (consider the cost, not whether the demands are achieved)
Get a better balance of work and leisure	View a situation with curiosity rather than with criticism	Manage disappointing results
Share a vulnerability with someone	Embrace and learn from mistakes rather than running from them	Resolve a conflict
Tune in and respond more to what your feelings are telling you	Take more pride in oneself (being a more respectful self-parent)	Strut
Be Silly or just take yourself less seriously	Smile at your reflection	Initiate plans
Try something new	Get Messy	Break a ritual
Get more sleep	Other	Other

Possible Suggestions:	My Plan:
☐ Positive attention when takes a step toward behavior ☐ One-on-one time outside of eating disorder stuff ☐ Earning a logical privilege given increased health ☐ Praise and STOP – no BUTS ☐ Role Model Behavior Yourself ☐ Open the door for a discussion ☐ Set a limit ☐ Offer to teach ☐ Other	

Heathy Coping Strategy I will Role Model this week.

Possible Suggestions:	My Plan:
☐ Delegate something. ☐ Say 'no' to some things. ☐ Be honest with my feelings. ☐ Express my feelings when not on the wave. ☐ Ask for help. ☐ Set healthy limits between my needs and those of others. ☐ Listen with full attention. ☐ Praise and STOP. ☐ Say "I'm sorry" with no excuses. ☐ Allow family members to make mistakes Without jumping in. ☐ Be consistent. ☐ Address negative self-talk. ☐ Be reliable.	

Self-care Strategy I will implement this week

Possible Suggestions:	My Plan:
☐ Make regular mealtimes a priority. ☐ Set a regular bedtime. ☐ Learn a new hobby. ☐ Spend some time with my friends. ☐ Spend time ALONE with my spouse. ☐ Set a regular time I stop work each day. ☐ Take weekends off. ☐ Buy something for myself. ☐ Exercise in a MODERATE manner. ☐ Take pride in my physical appearance.	No lame excuses!!

TIP OF THE WEEK: Symptoms are signs there is a problem that needs solving.

CHAPTER EIGHT: The Power of Example

Where You Are

- ✓ You have finished your first step. You have learned more about the program.

- ✓ You have learned more about the stages of parenting and how eating disorders take your child off the path of healthy growth.

- ✓ You have learned about strategies of parenting and emotion regulation that can help you be more effective in your role.

- ✓ You have learned about healthy nutrition and how this gets confused by your child's disorder.

- ✓ You have learned about behavior and he factors that keep it going.

- ✓ You have learned about the barriers that get in the way of behavior change.

Congratulations!!

You are now a key player in your child's treatment team.

Key Messages

It's a process: try, tweak, learn, grow.

"Self-parenting" is a necessary step for "other parenting."

Stay off the WAVE.

Remain genuine.

Topic: The Journey

Now it's time for the step that can bring annoyance and fear to the hearts of all parents – taking a look at your own behavior. This is extremely important. Fortunately or unfortunately, your children are smart. If we teach them to do one thing, then we do another, they are going to greatly question the wisdom of our advice (as well they should). In contrast, if we are advising our children while WE are taking steps to do these same things ourselves, then our child is more likely to want to engage in these behaviors too! In addition, it is much EASIER to learn a new skill if someone else is doing it as well. Thus, our theme is this:

"Be as you want your child to be."

Why is caring for yourself important?

Consider our magical formula:

Step One	You treat yourself well
Step Two	Your needs are being met, so your anxiety decreases and your ability to handle life increases.
Step Three	You give off this positive "karma" that comes from individuals who feel connected and cared for by themselves.
Step Four	Others start to respond more positively to you because this positive karma is very magnetizing – low anxiety, "together" people are quite attractive!
Step Five	Life seems more pleasant as there seems to be more positive around you.
Step Six	Your child looks at your example and thinks, "Hmm, s/he seems to have it all together", and wants that for herself.
Step Seven	**LIFE IMPROVES.....**

Oh my gosh!! I have so much to do. I don't know how I am going to get it done. Guess there's no sleep for me tonight. That's the price I pay for having so many people need me.

Stressed Out Person

It will get done. Just not today. Today I want to spend time with my family. All these things can wait till tomorrow. Or the next day.

Cool as a Cucumber Person

Ready to jump in?   If you think this makes sense, that setting a good example is important, and you are ready to go ahead, keep reading. If instead, you find yourself thinking of a million excuses, then skip to the "pep talk" on page 130 and then, hopefully, you'll come right back!

You, the Honored Guest

Our goal is to have you treat yourself with respect, as if you were your own best friend. Some people simply do not know where to begin in becoming their own best friend. Even more complicated, some people don't even know what their needs are. If this sounds like you, this chapter will be very important in helping you to define your goals and values.

Step One. Treat yourself as you would an honored guest

Picture this: The person you most admire in the entire world is coming to stay in your home. This famous celebrity, world leader, writer is to be a guest in your home for an extended period of time. Think about the preparations you would make and the things you would do to prepare for this honored guest.

When I have surveyed people regarding what they would do, these are some examples of responses that I have received:

To Do List

- *Clean the house*
- *Buy favorite foods*
- *Make something special*
- *Look at entertainment section for fun things to do*
- *Plan some fun activities*
- *Get some flowers*
- *Take time off*
- *Buy a bottle of good wine*

Think about the **PROCESS** that went into deciding what you would do. Chances are, you thought about your guest and you put yourself in his or her shoes. You imagined what he/she would like to experience when he/she visited. You thought about the things that would make your guest feel cared for and pampered.

This is the goal that we are aiming for. We want you to STOP and REFLECT about what YOU would like and what YOU would appreciate in the moment. This is about directing some of your attention INWARD, asking yourself what you NEED and WANT, RESPECTING THAT NEED OR WANT, and taking steps to meet that need. This is about learning to dance with yourself.

Sounds simple, huh? We know that putting it into practice is a whole different matter.

> **WE WANT YOU TO LEARN TO DANCE WITH YOURSELF,**
> - to check in with yourself,
> - to be in sync with your needs,
> - to be flexible in your steps when your body tells you a different direction,
> - to be a firm and supportive instructor.

To help you understand and appreciate what we are aiming for, we want to introduce you to a paradigm shift. This is a new way of looking at yourself and the world that we have been hinting at, and that we will explain more fully. We will keep referring to this philosophy throughout the remainder of this program.

Step Two: The Paradigm Shift

Our first step in achieving this dance with ourselves is to adjust our focus a bit; from an outcome focus to a balanced process focus.

What is an "outcome-focused" perspective?

Put simply, if we view life as a journey, then an "outcome" focus to life concentrates exclusively on where we end up. "Outcome" focused people just concentrate on the end of the road – how soon they will get there, the importance of where they are going, and after they get there, where they are going next.

We live in an outcome focused society. We focus our energy and our interest on the end results of our efforts and tend to neglect or ignore the process or experiences that we go through to achieve these outcomes. Examples of outcomes include the grades we receive, the amount of money we make, and the number of possessions we own. Why are so many people focused on outcome? Well, first consider the positives.

Positives of an Exclusive Outcome Focus

1. It makes things very simple. You either achieve the outcome or you fail.

2. Everybody else is doing it so you fit right in.

3. It feels really good when you achieve your outcome focused goal.

4. You often get rewarded for achieving an outcome focused goal.

5. It *appears* to make it more likely to achieve the goal, since all your energy is devoted to it.

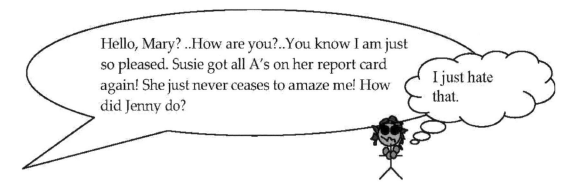

An exclusive outcome-focus emphasizes:

The grades you earn, class ranking, the money you could earn from a job, the status of a college choice, the number of possessions you own, the label of your clothes, the status of your parents, choosing friends based on influence or popularity, an ideal body type an ideal weight.

Negatives of an Exclusive Outcome Focus

1. It creates a non-cooperative, competitive environment.
2. You never stop and smell the roses and benefit from your experiences along the way.
3. Learning new ways is limited.
4. It can take the joy out of doing anything.
5. Many individuals do not feel satisfied even when they achieve the outcome since the next step is right around the corner.
6. It can feel empty when you get there. Since it is all you've focused on, when you finally achieve the goal, you can be left with an empty "now what?" feeling.
7. It can actually impair your ability to achieve the goal since you get so nervous by placing such importance on it.
8. You may be afraid to try new things since new experiences are associated with initial trial and error.

The Alternative is "A Balanced Process Perspective"

We would like you to consider the wisdom of another perspective: a process perspective. Let's go back to our journey. Unlike "outcome-folks," a Process person takes a look around where he is at each stage of the journey.

Process is...... "Hmm, what strengths brought me here? How can I use these strengths for my next step?"

Process is...... "Hmm, look at that next side road. That road may suit my values better."

Process is....... "Hmm, it sure is nice right here. Maybe I should stay here for a little bit."

Process is......

- learning with an open mind – you are willing to try new ways of doing things
- personal style – you think about your body and your personal tastes and you dress to suit you
- personal values – you check in with yourself and make sure your actions match YOUR values, not another's
- enjoyment – you have fun
- meaning – you see the value in quality conversations in the moment, time for yourself, silence
- sharing – you are willing to teach as well as to learn
- valuing others for their talents – you admire people and try to learn from them
- willingness to accept mistakes – how can you learn otherwise?
- flexibility – you are willing to change course

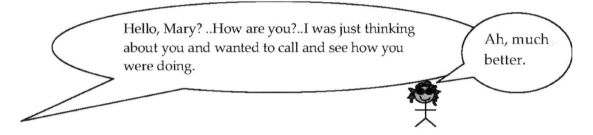

The benefits of a "process" based focus are:

1. You are in the moment rather than worrying about what will happen. This allows you to be more effective in the moment and may result in a positive change to "what would have happened."

2. Your focus is on appreciating the current decision and learning from it, rather than dwelling on the decisions you "could have made."

3. You are descriptive rather than critical.

4. You are accepting of the circumstances that placed you in your current situation rather than regretting where you "could be" had things turned out differently.

5. You use current experiences to learn, and apply what you have learned to the current situation and the one to follow.

6. You are vibrantly alive.

7. Your mind is open to learning without fear.

8. You can try new things without fearing mistakes as "mistakes" are nonexistent, just opportunities for learning.

9. You are open to alternatives.

✿ Perfectionist's Corner ✿

Perfectionist: Get real. That sound ideal, but this is the real world we're talking about. Grades, where people go to college – these things matter.

Voice of Reason: Yes and no. Stop a minute and think about truly successful people you know. Truly successful. People who seem to experience joy out of their work and their family. People who have a creative spark. I don't dispute that they have achieved great outcomes. They didn't FOCUS on the outcomes, they focused on the JOURNEY. By doing so, their mind was free to find the right path for them and thus, they were successful. I have seen this in action clinically and research supports it.   I can't but believe this is true.

Perfectionist: But people who keep their eyes focused on the goals and don't let anything get in their way are more likely to achieve the goal

Voice of Reason: Actually, a large body of research demonstrates the exact opposite. Putting such exclusive emphasis on an outcome increases anxiety and tension towards achieving the goal. Although a little bit of anxiety can spur us to work harder, too much actually impedes our performance. In addition, research shows that creativity and problem-solving are enhanced by positive moods. Such creative exploration helps us learn new strategies that strengthen our ability to learn more in the future!

Our goal is balance. As you will see, an exclusive "outcome focus" is the cornerstone of a competitive environment that breeds dissatisfaction with ourselves and others and helps to foster attitudes that lead to eating disorder development. Shifting to a process or experientially based focus can create a fertile environment for learning, questioning, self-acceptance, happiness, and creative thought. Such an environment may go far in helping to foster happiness in you and in your family.

> **TIP BOX**
>
> Our goal is balance.   We use an outcome to choose our INITIAL path and then let the joy and experience of the journey guide and shape the path. Where will we end up? We have a reasonable idea but, ultimately, we'll see when we get there!

Now, don't misunderstand, there is a need for outcomes. Outcomes help us to choose a certain path and help to direct our actions. The problem comes when we **exclusively** focus on outcomes. When we do so, several unfortunate consequences may occur.

Step Three: Applying a Process Perspective to Ourselves

So how do we apply this philosophy to ourselves so we can begin the process of treating ourselves as an honored guest? Let's compare the two.

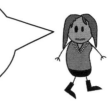

Look, I am convinced. This just feels right to me. Would you mind speaking to all the other people in my neighborhood and at my school? The hard part is sticking to this when everyone else is warped.

I'll touch on this in the question and answer section.

Outcome Focus

An outcome-focused approach to OURSELF involves comparing who we are in the current moment to an IDEAL self and focuses on how far we have to go to be that "IDEAL", a standard that is usually unattainable. If this weren't bad enough (always falling short), the TONE of this comparison is an added problem. An outcome focus is usually a shameful and guilty focus. Rather than focus on who we ARE, an outcome takes a blaming and shameful stance regarding any discrepancy between who you ARE and who you SHOULD be. Sadly, often we get so discouraged by this huge discrepancy, we lose all motivation to improve anything. It seems we'll never reach the goal, so why bother trying? When we're in this state of mind, the thought of treating oneself as an honored guest is often met with "Well, when I am at my ideal, then I'll want to treat myself as an honored guest. Until then, where I am is intolerable." Or "How can I accept myself, when I am like this??"

Process Focus

Process focuses on the NOW. It is an "OK, this is what I have. What can I work on? What do I have to work on accepting? What are my strengths and how do I maximize those? What are my weaknesses and how do I improve those?" In other words, it is acceptance of yourself in the now with an eye on where you would like to head. It is enjoying where you find yourself on the journey, not despairing because you haven't arrived yet.

General Guidelines of a Process Focus towards Yourself

1. Check in with yourself, <u>every day</u>.
Try to begin and end your day with a "check-in." It also would be a wise idea to buy a pack of stickers and put them in random places where you will see them throughout the day. Whenever you see one, it is a cue to check in and have a good conversation.   "Hello, Self. How are you feeling?"

2. <u>Accept</u> **how you feel and how you are.** "Tired! Well, we need to look at your bedtimes..."

3. <u>Meet</u> **your needs, <u>don't</u> judge them.**

Hungry? EAT. Don't criticize your hunger. Tired?   Make time for more rest. Don't judge your energy level. Sad?   Sadness can be a symptom of loss, a sign that you need more tender loving care, a sign of loneliness....<u>Investigate</u> what your sadness is telling you using the wave skills you have learned and meet that need. Mad? Same principle. Investigate what made you angry and address the source in an appropriate way.

4. **Always try to <u>learn</u> more about yourself. Expand your horizons. Look for new opportunities. Keep your eyes open.**
"Yes, I'd like to try that painting class. I'm not sure if I'd enjoy art or not."

2.   **Accept yourself completely both as you are now and as a <u>permanent</u> work in progress.**

Remember to use life as an opportunity to learn, not as something which you win or lose.

SELF-ASSESSMENT

What we are going to do in the next section is to think about various aspects of your life that are very important – how you care for yourself, how you balance your time, how you feel about the way you look, etc. We will compare what an outcome oriented approach relative to a process-oriented approach would look like in each area.

For each area, we want you to take a minute to think about yourself. Where do you fit on this continuum? Is this an area you struggle with? Would you be comfortable if your child was exactly like you in this area? Are you treating yourself as an **honored guest?**

You may find as a result of this assessment that this is an area you could use a little work on. It is important to remember something – <u>we could all use work in these areas.</u>   If this is a problem area for you, make a note on the assessment part of each chapter. To give you some ideas regarding how you would begin to address these areas, each chapter has a suggestion box of possible goals. As we complete our homework for the remainder of this program, we will use these goals as guides for what to work on.

TIP BOX

Here are some important things to keep in mind as you write these goals.

1. Don't panic. We will not work on all these goals this week. Rather, these goals will help to shape what we work on in ourselves throughout the rest of this program. We are always, for the rest of our lives, a work in progress. Hopefully we are always striving to learn more about ourselves and to grow. Setting goals is a part of this process -as is being open to changing the goals as we change.

2. We will take baby steps. Each time we approach a goal, we will break it down into manageable pieces that you think you can handle.

3. Don't be afraid to write down goals even if the thought of achieving them seems impossible. Part of our task through this group is to raise your confidence that you can achieve these goals. For now, just dream. We'll get there.

Barriers: The Pep Talk

Learning how to take good care of yourself, while balancing all your other responsibilities, is extremely challenging. As tough as it is, certain beliefs that we have may make this task seem overwhelming or unnecessary. Let's consider a few of those beliefs and how we can help you to work through them so that taking care of yourself doesn't become a chore or a hassle, but rather, something that actually makes life more enjoyable.

First, don't forget our "magical" formula.

MAGICAL FORMULA

Start with some advice.
1. You advise your child to care of herself. Add in some role modeling.
2. You start taking better care of yourself. Mix in your child's intelligence.
3. Your child sees you following your own advice and begins to take your advice more seriously.
4. Your child sees you getting happier and less stressed as you take better care of yourself. Your child REALLY starts understanding the value of your advice by watching the positive effect on you. Add some good reasoning.
5. Your child starts taking better care of herself.
6. You feel better. Your child feels better.
7. You can both handle stress better because you feel better. And you end up with........

Things that used to bother you no longer do because you can handle stress better.

LIFE GETS BETTER!

Second, consider these **"BELIEF BARRIERS"**

What follows are some examples of beliefs that may make it more difficult for you to care for yourself. We offer some thoughts about these beliefs. As you read through this, think about your own beliefs that may get in the way.

The belief: I am too busy to set aside time for myself or to worry about myself.

The challenge: Well, if it's any comfort, this is our most popular excuse. Actually, the exact opposite is true. If you take the time to care for yourself, you are more efficient so things take less time (and are easier to deal with!). Promise.

The belief: I don't deserve to take care of myself.

The challenge: THIS is a biggie. A belief like this stems from one's learning history. Somewhere along the way, you picked up the notion that you don't deserve to be cared for. This is a belief that you will have to attack bit by bit as you go through these steps - particularly the one on perfectionism. One of the principles that we try to teach you, so you can convey this message to your child, is that people are special just because. There is no universal grading system that makes one person more special than another. Rather, we all are a unique combination of our beliefs, our interests, our values, our personality, etc. In short, we are all special. If you struggle with this belief, it is important that you give it some serious thought. Your child struggles with this a lot, in all probability. Many individuals with eating disorders believe that the only thing that makes you special is what you DO. This is a losing proposition, because you know what, we can always do more. And, someone will always do it better. Besides, do what? What is important for one person may not be important for another. It makes much more sense to value each individual for their individuality. Doesn't it? We all deserve to be taken care of.

If this is a belief that you struggle with, we don't expect it to change overnight. However, in the meantime, we suggest you think about "faking it until you make it." Your child needs you to be a positive role model. If at this point you cannot do it for yourself, think about whether you can take some steps in the interest of your child.

The belief: Man, this will take a lot of work, and frankly, this disorder has already knocked the wind out of my sails. I am tired.

The challenge: I can't challenge that. Children are challenging and tiring and rewarding and wonderful, all at the same time (O.K., nearly the same time). After having done this program for many years and watched families go through, I can't tell you it is not tiring, but I can tell you the rewards are great. Through this process, both you and your child will grow as individuals and feel more secure in your footing, balanced in your values, closer in your relationships, and will live more genuine lives. As with anything, **you will get out of this program what you put it in. Good things are worth fighting for.**

The belief: My child is not living at home. Can I really make a difference?

The challenge: Yes. I work with many adult patients and, I can tell you, the influence of their parents' opinions continues to weigh greatly with them. I cannot think of anything more powerful to model than the willingness to embrace and acknowledge mistakes and a willingness to do things differently.

The patients I work with are so exceedingly pleased, amazed, relieved, excited, when their parents are striving to make the same changes they are. Just like you may wish I could change all your neighbors, it is easier to change when the whole family is working, no matter where everyone lives. Just make sure you talk about the changes.

Try writing some of your own belief barriers that are more individualized to your unique circumstances.

☐ I am too busy.

☐ I am not important enough.

☐ I am not sure it will help.

Key Points

Let's summarize what we have learned about parenting and eating disorders. In the next chapter, we'll explain what the experience of an eating disorder is like for your child and how an "Off the C.U.F.F." approach can make it easier for both you and your child to manage the disorder.

- The main goal of parenting is for your child to learn to be a kind and supportive parent for him or herself.
- Children with an eating disorder have yet to internalize this parent. I always worry how some parents will read this. Instead they have internalized a cruel, unforgiving parent, an eating disorder.
- Their eating disorder serves as a coping strategy. We need to figure out how their disorder helps them cope so we can teach them healthier strategies.
- You have already done this.
- Talk is cheap. The best way for your children to learn healthy strategies is for you to role model them (it's good for you too).
- Taking care of yourself is an extremely important part of this program: it communicates to your child that this is important, is shows your child how to do it, and you are worth it!

Weekly Goals

We'll stick to the usual homework sheet. However, we have an interesting exercise for you to try. Try asking your child what he or she thinks your values are. It may make for an interesting conversation.

Questions and Answers

Q: How can I implement a process focus when the whole world is outcome focused and everyone else keeps forcing the issue?

A: Believe it or not, the shift is a lot easier than you realize. In their hearts, most parents believe in the values inherent in a "process" approach. They are just afraid. They want their children to be accepted and to be financially secure. They are afraid that an outcome focus is necessary to achieve this. It isn't.

You can't control other people. What you can control is your own behavior when you interact with others. Others choose how they respond. Your job is not to proselytize. Just be true to your values. Here's an example:

Neighbor: Did your son do okay on the end-of-year tests? I am so relieved my child scored at the top of the class again.

You: **(strategy-a subtle shift in conversation topic to process without person realizing it).** You know, I am so frustrated by this end-of-year testing. The quality of education is going downhill since the emphasis is so placed on these tests and not on valuable learning experiences. I have seen my child's love of school gradually diminishing and I am so saddened by this. We have to do something.

Neighbor: You know you're right! I think it's awful. We should both go to the next school board meeting.

Others will shift easier than you think. They want to. They are just afraid.

Wisdom of the Week: My Gift to Myself

Our gift to ourselves this week is to appreciate the value of children's books. Thus, we give you a quote from one of our favorite books, *The Little Prince* by Antoine de Saint-Exupery. Hopefully you will have a whole new appreciation of the meaning of this quote after this most recent step.

"My drawing was not a picture of a hat. It was a picture of a boa constrictor digesting an elephant…In the course of this life I have had a great many encounters with a great many people who have been concerned with matters of consequence. I have lived a great deal among grown-ups. I have seen them intimately, close at hand. And that hasn't much improved my opinion of them. Whenever I met one of them who seemed to me at all clear-sighted, I tried the experiment of showing him my Drawing Number One, which I have always kept. I would try to find out, so, if this was a person of true understanding. But, whoever it was, he, or she, would always say: 'That is a hat.' Then I would never talk to that person about boa constrictors, or primeval forests, or stars. I would bring myself down to his level. I would talk to him about bridge, and golf, and politics, and neckties. And the grown-up would be greatly pleased to have met such a sensible man."

Don't you just love that? Get's to the point doesn't it. Process is about imagination, creativity, and experience.

C'mon. Pull out a children's book. You know you want to.

Date:

Remember our key guidelines
It's a process! Try, tweak, grow and learn.
Self-parenting: a necessary prerequisite for other parenting.
Learn how to SURF The WAVE!
Remain genuine.

Unhealthy or unhelpful behavior I will discuss WITH my child this week and our plan to address it.

Eats too little	Eats too little variety	Exercises too much
Throws up after meals	Doesn't get enough sleep	Doesn't set limits
Abuses laxatives	Engages in self-harm	Other

Possible Suggestions of How to Address:
☐ Ignore it
☐ Have a discussion about needed change in behavior
 (discuss a future, necessary, logical consequence given the severity of the behavior)
☐ Implement a logical consequence (reminding your child of the importance of health before anything)
☐ Appeal to your child's inner wisdom (have a discussion with your child about what you have observed, why you are concerned, the change in behavior expected)
☐ Reverse Time-Out (you leave)
☐ Group Time-Out (everyone leaves for 10 minutes)
☐ Regrouping (family meeting to get out of power struggle)
☐ Humor

My Plan:

Would a discussion be a good idea?

Heathy Coping Strategy I will address with my child this week and my plan to address it.

Express negative emotions effectively	Ask for more help	Set more limits (cut down study time, set a regular bedtime, cut out an activity)
Express an opinion- even if someone may disagree	Be more considerate of others	Place more realistic demands on oneself (consider the cost, not whether the demands are achieved)
Get a better balance of work and leisure	View a situation with curiosity rather than with criticism	Manage disappointing results
Share a vulnerability with someone	Embrace and learn from mistakes rather than running from them	Resolve a conflict
Tune in and respond more to what your feelings are telling you	Take more pride in oneself (being a more respectful self-parent)	Strut
Be Silly or just take yourself less seriously	Smile at your reflection	Initiate plans
Try something new	Get Messy	Break a ritual
Get more sleep	Other	Other

Possible Suggestions:	**My Plan:**
☐ Positive attention when takes a step toward behavior ☐ One-on-one time outside of eating disorder stuff ☐ Earning a logical privilege given increased health ☐ Praise and STOP – no BUTS ☐ Role Model Behavior Yourself ☐ Open the door for a discussion ☐ Set a limit ☐ Offer to teach ☐ Other	

Heathy Coping Strategy I will Role Model this week.

Possible Suggestions:	**My Plan:**
☐ Delegate something. ☐ Say 'no' to some things. ☐ Be honest with my feelings. ☐ Express my feelings when not on the wave. ☐ Ask for help. ☐ Set healthy limits between my needs and those of others. ☐ Listen with full attention. ☐ Praise and STOP. ☐ Say "I'm sorry" with no excuses. ☐ Allow family members to make mistakes without jumping in. ☐ Be consistent. ☐ Address negative self-talk. ☐ Be reliable.	

Self-care Strategy I will implement this week

Possible Suggestions:	**My Plan:**
☐ Make regular mealtimes a priority. ☐ Set a regular bedtime. ☐ Learn a new hobby. ☐ Spend some time with my friends. ☐ Spend time ALONE with my spouse. ☐ Set a regular time I stop work each day. ☐ Take weekends off. ☐ Buy something for myself. ☐ Exercise in a MODERATE manner. ☐ Take pride in my physical appearance.	No lame excuses!!

TIP OF THE WEEK: Respect yourself.

CHAPTER NINE: Process and You

Where You Are

- ✓ You have finished your first step. You have learned more about the program.

- ✓ You have learned more about the stages of parenting and how eating disorders take your child off the path of healthy growth.

- ✓ You have learned about strategies of parenting and emotion regulation that can help you be more effective in your role.

- ✓ You have learned about healthy nutrition and how this gets confused by your child's disorder.

- ✓ You have learned about behavior and he factors that keep it going.

- ✓ You have learned about the barriers that get in the way of behavior change.

- ✓ You have been introduced to our experiential, process approach to life.

Congratulations!!

You'll soon be ready to take your show on the road.

Key Messages

It's a process: try, tweak, learn, grow.

"Self-parenting" is a necessary step for "other parenting."

Stay off the WAVE.

Remain genuine.

Topic: Applying a Process Approach

In this chapter, we will take our process approach and apply it to discrete areas in your life: your hunger and appetite, your view of your own physical appearance, your balance between your behaviors and your values, and your rest. These are changes that we want your child to be able to make. We want you to understand how this process comes about so you can be a wise and believable teacher.

We also want you to think about this next paragraph very carefully.

Important paragraph you need to pay attention to.

Remember in the first few chapters when we discussed Maslow's hierarchy of needs and the importance of meeting those needs? Well, it is time to think about this again. Listening and responding to your own needs forms the foundation of crucial aspects of identity and personal development: self-knowledge, self-trust, and self-direction. "Dancing with your body", i.e. listening to what your body is telling you and responding to those needs in a healthy manner, helps you get to know yourself. You learn about your own hunger patterns. You learn about your energy level. You learn the "type of person" you are. This back and forth dance, listening and responding, is the essence of "self-parenting" and, as we have learned, parents who reliably set healthy limits and meet their child's needs earns their child's trust. By analogy, self-parenting brings self-trust. Self-knowledge and self-trust, in turn, bring self-confidence, something your child is probably greatly struggling with. If you understand this process, you'll be a real help.

Although we have broken this process of self-knowledge into very discreet steps that may seem trivial to you, the importance of this chapter cannot be overemphasized. There, I'm finished. I needed to get that out.

Step 1: Hunger

What would a process vs. outcome approach to your own hunger and eating patterns look like? Time for a self-check. See what you find out.

Outcome Approach
Check the things you currently do.
☐   You picture an ideal way to eat and feel like a failure whenever you don't eat in that manner.
☐   You eat according to rule, not according to taste or hunger.
☐   You neglect hunger and regular eating if it interferes with your chosen outcome-focus goal of the moment.
☐   You criticize your hunger or are afraid of your hunger.

Process Approach
Check the things from which you would benefit.

☐ You make the act of eating an example of dancing with yourself.
- You start off the meal checking in with yourself to see how hungry you are.
- You start eating, SLOWLY (not eating disorder slowly, just slowly).
- During the meal, you check in with yourself to gage your hunger.
- You let feelings of fullness decide when you are finished with the meal.

It is this back-and-forth process with your body during a meal that is the "dance of eating." *Ah, my stomach is telling me I'm done. Time to stop. This was so delicious that I'll wrap up the rest and have more tomorrow or for dinner.*

☐ You try to learn more about your hunger by paying attention to your personal hunger patterns. *Are you hungrier at night? In the morning? Do you like salty in the morning and sweet in the evening?*

☐ You try to distinguish emotional hunger (e.g. stress eating) from biological hunger (my body is telling me it needs food) and work on different strategies to manage emotions than using food. *Hmmm. I know I am not really hungry. Just lonely. I think I'll pick up the phone.*

☐ You recognize that you are human. Thus, sometimes you will eat when you are not hungry (to celebrate, because the food tastes really good, etc.) You accept this as part of your humanness and move on. *What an amazing experience this restaurant it. I want to try one of their desserts as part of the joy of this moment.*

☐ You are alert for patterns of an unhealthy use of food (e.g., eating for sadness every once in a while is human, eating every time we are sad is a pattern) and start to address the patterns. *Hmm, every time I meet with my boss at work, I get upset and skip lunch. I need to not let that jerk get the best of me and go talk to a colleague instead and have a lovely lunch with her on my boss's expense card. (kidding)*

☐ You make mealtimes a priority. Because you believe in the importance of self-trust, you know you need to protect your own basic needs to earn your own trust of yourself. You put other things aside. *No, sorry. I have another "lunch" meeting at 12, but I can meet at 1pm.*

☐ You have a balanced attitude towards toward (you make healthy good choices while allowing treats you enjoy. *Balance = healthy fruits and vegetables + whole grains + special treats + low-fat protein.*

☐ You don't make food and eating a moral issue by accepting your hunger rather than judging it. *Boy, I'm hungry today! I feel like that sandwich was just an appetizer.*

☐ You create a calm, relaxing and peaceful environment around mealtimes. *Honey, if you wouldn't mind turning off that wrestling match while we eat, I would greatly appreciate it.*

Process Approach, cont'd.

Check the things from which you would benefit.

☐ You don't multi-task. You just eat. Slowly. *No sir, I didn't realize I had gotten a tuna salad stain on the report I gave you.*

☐ You enjoy the spiritual and special nature of eating with others and use that time to converse and share good food – not to watch television or argue or bring in outcome-focused topics. *Actually dear, I don't now is the time to discuss what went wrong with our sex life. Let's enjoy this time and save that until later. Ideally, when our parents are not present.*

For example, Doris Denial basically is not listening to herself. She has figured out a lifestyle that "suits her needs." She eats on the run, has sporadic meals or no meals depending on her work schedule, and is trying the latest diet of the month. Sure, she binge eats every night, but she deserves it, she works hard all day.

Think about these different approaches and your current attitude toward your own hunger and eating. From your assessment, write down some goals on your goal sheet. For each goal, write down a baby step that would represent one step closer to achieving that goal, but at a pace that is reasonable. If you need some suggestions, look at the suggestion box below.

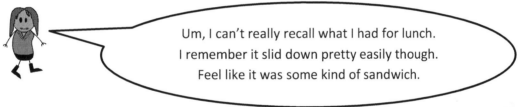

Um, I can't really recall what I had for lunch.
I remember it slid down pretty easily though.
Feel like it was some kind of sandwich.

YOUR TURN

For each goal, write down a baby step that would represent one step closer to achieving that goal, but at a pace that is reasonable. If you need some suggestions, look at the suggestion box below.

SUGGESTION BOX

GOALS (baby steps to reach these goals)

Take time for breakfast. *For 2 days this week I will go to bed an hour earlier so I can get up earlier and have breakfast.*

Don't do other things while I eat. *For 2 days this week, I will have my lunch after the rush hour down in my office cafeteria and sit outside and eat by myself.*

Clear off the kitchen table. *Buy an organizer for the kitchen desk so I can begin the process of clearing.*

Eat slowly. *For 1meal each day, I will put my fork down in between bites*

Give myself a lunch break. *For 2 days this week, I will schedule a lunch break.*

Incorporate foods I've avoided in with foods I enjoy. *I will make a list of foods I am fearful of eating or that I associate with stress eating.*

SUGGESTION BOX (cont'd)

Make a few more family meals. *I will inform the family that Sunday will be a family meal.*
Stop throughout the meal to check in with my hunger. *For one meal each day, I will put down my fork and stop halfway through to check in with my hunger.*
Watch my negative self-talk during meals. *For one meal each day, I will challenge any negative self-talk that occurs during the meal.*

What have you learned?	
Write down 2 goals related to your hunger and the baby steps it will take to reach these goals.	
Goal #1:	**Goal #2:**
Baby steps to reach goal #1:	**Baby steps to reach goal #2:**
a)	**a)**
b)	**b)**
c)	**c)**

Step 2: Rest

Are you getting the hang of this? Let's try rest. First, a word on why rest is important. Rest is important. Without rest you would die. Rest decreases stress. Research suggests adequate rest may decrease stress eating. Learning occurs during sleep. Each day brings new experiences. Well, the new pathways formed in your brain keep re-firing and strengthening during sleep. Finally, sleeping is fun. Jumping into bed is fun. Napping is delightful. Getting out of bed? Not so fun.

Outcome Approach **Check the things you currently do.**	Process Approach **Check the things you need to work on.**
☐ You make a rule about the amount of sleep one "should" have and adhere to that rule.	☐ You find out how much sleep you need by listening to your body.
☐ You feel guilty if you sleep more than the allotted amount.	☐ You try to prioritize your sleep by stopping work at a reasonable time.
☐ You deem sleep as lazy and allow other activities to interfere with getting enough sleep.	☐ You establish a regular sleeping and winding down routing.
	☐ You allow yourself to sleep more when your body needs it.

SUGGESTION BOX

Goals - *baby steps to reach these goals.*

Figure out how much sleep my body needs. *This week, I will follow my usual behavior regarding sleep but will make some rating of my fatigue in the morning, afternoon and evening to see if tiredness seems to be a problem. WORD OF CAUTION: BE ALERT FOR ABUSE OF CAFFEINE OR OTHER STRATEGIES TO REDUCE FATIGUE.*

Set a regular sleeping schedule. *For two days this week, I will stop at a set time in the evening regardless of what I still have left to do.*

I will stop criticizing my sleep habits. *When I wake up in the morning, I will challenge the initial verbal abuse I give myself about pushing the snooze button.*

Get more sleep. *I will advance my bedtime by 15 minutes every night this week.*

What have you learned?	
Write down 2 goals related to your rest and the baby steps it will take to reach these goals.	
Goal #1:	**Goal #2:**
Baby steps to reach goal #1:	**Baby steps to reach goal #2:**
a)	a)
b)	b)
c)	c)

Step 3: Physical Appearance

The next area that we will address is physical appearance. Before we apply our process vs. outcome philosophy to this area, we would like to give you some background information on this topic since this is such an important issue for your child.

In this section, our focus is on helping you to develop or improve your evaluation of your own physical appearance and self-pride and to take steps to deemphasize the importance of physical appearance relative to other areas that make you who you "are."

You may be surprised that we are advising you to positively emphasize physical appearance. Given your child's fixation with the way he/she looks, you might expect us to say "don't talk about the way you look at all costs." Our emphasis is self-acceptance, self-comfort, and personal pride, which includes taking pride in one's appearance. Beauty, in turn, flows from these feelings. We hope to give a new understanding of physical appearance that you can embody in yourself in the hopes that these changes influence the attitude of your household towards re-conceptualizing true beauty.

Tip Box

Keep in mind that, for now, we are talking about YOUR relationship to YOUR appearance. The issue of physical appearance is currently fearful for your child, so with him or her we need to take baby steps. In the beginning stages of the illness, all talks of physical appearance are pretty much a "top of the wave" experience. As you have probably learned by now, you just can't say anything "right" when it comes to the physical appearance of your child.

Instead, a strategy you might consider is one like this: "Look, whenever you ask me for reassurance about your appearance or whenever I try to offer encouragement, we both get upset. I think this means that we're not ready for that yet. Let's just focus on your health and trust that healthy people become beautiful, in many, many ways. The next time you ask me about how you look, I am just going to say, "You will always be beautiful to me."

Do what works for you, but the main point is that questions about appearance are usually not asked when your child is in a calm state of mind and thus they are unlikely to use any response constructively. You're better off just refocusing attention.

A Philosophy of Beauty

Our outward appearance is our window to the outside world – the connection between what is going on inside of us and everything going on around us. However, it is actually not the nuances of this outside shell that are important (i.e. the number of gray hairs, the percentage of body fat, the shape of your face). Rather, your inner "aura", or inner self-comfort, colors your outside shell. This self-comfort contributes to your personal sense of beauty and to the perception others have of you as beautiful. Beauty truly flows from a deep sense of self-comfort other people can "sense" when they see you. Self-acceptance is magnetic. People are naturally attracted to people they perceive to be comfortable with themselves. Skeptical? Take a few moments to think about the people you are truly drawn to. Hmmm.

How does one arrive at this extreme level of self-acceptance and comfort? Well, of course we first return to our first key principle: trusting in the process and be willing to try, tweak, learn, and grow. However, we'll give you some starting steps.

1) Figure out from where you are starting. Take several minutes to think about your relationship with your own appearance. What happens when you look in the mirror? Do you experience a sense of satisfaction and comfort, or, in fact, do you owe yourself an apology? You may need to start off by clearing the slate, apologizing to yourself for being such a jerk, and starting anew. We could always use more practice with "I'm sorry, self."

2) Take note of the story told by your body. Your body reflects the journey of your life so far. Every part of your body conveys your own unique history. Hopefully this will help you put things in a different perspective to think of "character-building" traits rather than good or bad features. Our individual histories are fascinating and our bodies have been through it all with us.

3) Next, step back and take an inventory of "what you've got". Your inventory is descriptive not judgmental.   Pretend you are describing yourself to a police artist who needs to sketch an image of you for an investigation. Stick to facts. A police artist can't draw "an ugly mouth" but he can draw a thick upper lip.

4) Think about the aspects of your appearance you like. Take steps to accentuate those.

5) Think about the aspects of your appearance that you would change if provided the opportunity. Decide what aspects of those factors you have legitimate control over, and take steps to bolster those aspects. However, take steps towards enhancement out of personal pride, rather than guilt and shame. Work on accepting those things you cannot change as a unique part of you.

It might look something like this:

"Hello self. Time for an honest look. See this scar? Well, I got this that time I tripped while trying to help my dad wash the car. My stomach? Well, some reflects my first pregnancy, some my second pregnancy, and some came with menopause. I have green eyes, hair that is 35%, OK, 50% gray, and wrinkles around the corner of my eyes. I love my mouth and smile. I would switch out my nose if a fairy gave me a wish so I'll just work with it. It does have character. My shoulders slump so I can do something about that. I would like to have more muscular legs and can do something about that as well."

Tip Box

1. You start with self-acceptance. When you feel comfortable with yourself, you want to do nice things for yourself and take better care of yourself.
2. With this self-comfort and self-pride, you exude a positive aura.
3. People sense this aura and respond to you positively.
4. This positive interconnection generates more good feelings.
5. Your child senses your self-comfort and, suddenly, your advice carries more weight.

Many individuals have this formula mixed up. They think if they work on improving their outward appearance, they will feel more attractive. It makes sense that people would think this way. This is what we are told in media messages, advertisements, etc. In fact, it is not an exaggeration to say that we are bombarded with these messages constantly. However, if you think about it, this formula does not make sense. Our outward shell fluctuates throughout the day. One minute your hair is one way, your makeup another, etc. If our attractiveness were contingent on that shell, we would have to check the mirror every five minutes to make sure "all was well." Every day would be an agonizing roller coaster ride. One minute you feel attractive, the next minute you don't.   HOW EXHAUSTING!!!

However, self-pride is stable. If we regard ourselves as attractive and exude self-respect and self-pride, others will regard us as more attractive. Instead, if physical appearance is an aura that you give off internally, the general sense that "You know what, I like myself, and I look good," then this feeling would remain stable throughout the day. Makes sense doesn't it?

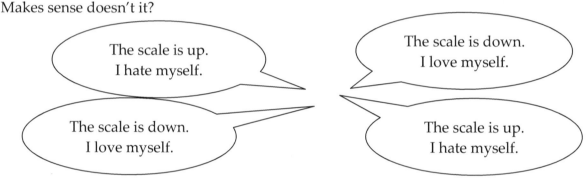

Physical Appearance and Your Children

So what about your child's attitudes and experiences regarding physical appearance? Well, often individuals with eating disorders have two fundamental problems when it comes to physical appearance:

Problem #1: They are dissatisfied with their current appearance.

Fortunately, the strategies we have been discussing regarding our comfort with our own physical appearance apply to your child as well. Thus, it is important to consider your own struggles with these issues to truly serve as a guide for your child. Ideally, we hope you can help each other become more comfortable with yourselves and take pride in the way you look.

Problem #2: They overemphasize the importance of physical appearance in relation to who they are as people.

Your child may have an additional difficulty, however. Individuals with eating disorders tend to place extreme importance on physical appearance in determining who they are as a person. How we define ourselves has important bearing on our happiness.

We will speak a great deal more about this when we talk about perfectionism. For now, it is important to understand a few key points.

Factors that Make People Unique

There is a difference between what we do and who we are. People get into trouble and often feel badly about themselves (or just fleetingly good) when they equate these two things. Who we are is a special combination of our personality traits, our beliefs, our values, our bizarre quirks, our interests, our habits the list goes on and on. Although we all grow and change as human beings, this change fluctuates around a stable core (our true self) that is consistent across situations and people. Otherwise, we would feel quite artificial, wouldn't we?

This self-definition is extremely different than an "outcome-based" self-definition. Outcome-focused individuals believe that self-definition is based on transitory achievements. The problem is, however, that transitory fluctuations do not really provide a stable sense of self. Rather, it is our unique core that defines who we are. Often individuals with an eating disorder have a very narrow definition of what makes a person special – they think it is all about the way they look. For example, if the pie chart below represented the different aspects of an individual, and the size of each slice represented the degree of importance of each facet of that individual, then an individual with an eating disorder may have a pie chart that looked like this.

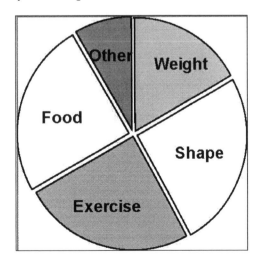

Instead, people are actually more complicated than this.

A healthy self-definition might look something like the pie chart below.

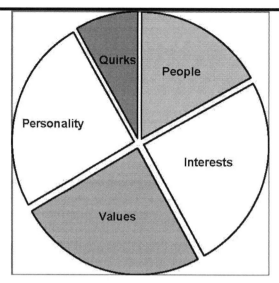

Now it's your turn! Let's relate what we have talked about regarding physical appearance into our "process vs. outcome" philosophy and start exploring the way in which you regard your own physical appearance. For the goals we set for this area, we will suggest some ways to help both you and your child with these areas.

Outcome Approach
Check the things you currently do.
☐ You compare yourself to a physical ideal and beat yourself up for not looking like that ideal.
☐ You refrain from taking pride in your appearance until you get to a certain weight.
☐ You restrict your activities if you feel you don't look "right".
☐ You criticize your physical appearance.

Process Approach
Check the things you currently do.
☐ You work on accepting the way you look now rather than waiting for an ideal weight or body shape in order to flaunt your style.
☐ You differentiate what you have control over regarding your physical appearance versus what you need to work on accepting regarding the way you look. You spend your energy on the former rather than worrying about the latter.
☐ You accept what you can't change, and take pride in what you have.
☐ You refrain from making self-deprecating comments about your appearance.
☐ You explore your personal style.
☐ You accentuate your strengths.
☐ You exude confidence in your physical appearance via your body language.
☐ You do something kind to your body every day.
☐ You speak to yourself in a respectful manner.
☐ You view your body as reflection of your unique history and extension of yourself and treat it as an honored guest.

What do we mean by the things we need to work on accepting and those that we can work on? Well, we like common sense. If beauty flows from within, if one of our **key principles is "remaining genuine,"** and if our bodies tell the stories of our lives, then frankly, anything that wipes out this story is quite sad. In today's society, there are many options for changing our appearance, some that involve surgical alterations of the way our body looks. You need to decide what options are best for you, keeping with our process approach, and working on remaining genuine to ourselves and our loved ones. Here are some examples to think about.

Things I Need to Accept	Things I Can Work Out
Where I carry my weight	Haircut
My body shape	My style
My height	My posture
My hair texture	My body language
My eye color	My make-up
My complexion	Use of accessories
My face shape	My aura
My body type	Beliefs about my appearance

Tip Box
Strategies to Address a Negative View of Your Appearance

I will work on accepting myself. *I will take an inventory of my personal likes and dislikes regarding my appearance; I will choose one of the things that I like and will explore how to bring out that feature)*

I will choose an aspect that I am not comfortable with and will work on that *e.g. I am not comfortable with my sense of grace, so I will sign up for a yoga class.*

I will work on my physical strength. *Two days this week, I will try a weight lifting program.*

I will improve my body language. *I will put reminder cues all over the house. When I see them, it will serve as a reminder to walk taller.*

I will stop making critical comments toward my appearance. *For one hour each day, I will practice walking like "I got it all going on" and will say positive comments to myself about my appearance while I do this.*

I will go shopping. *I will go shopping with the intention of buying something that suits my style without regard to size and what I "should" be wearing.*

I will start swimming. I will try a new hairdo.

Tips to help with over-emphasizing the importance of physical appearance:

1) Take a look at your own pie chart. Could it use some diversification? Maybe you and your child could try something new together! Think of a new hobby you would like to try. Make a list of the steps it would take to get started. Pick a baby step to do this week.

2) Model a lack of regard about physical appearance. Try not to make comments on an individual's physical appearance but rather to emphasize the holistic sense of people that we have been talking about.

3) Model critical thinking regarding media messages about weight and appearance. Read a magazine with your child and discuss the way the media distorts images and gives false messages.

4) Help your child explore new interests for the right reasons – not because they **should** do them, but because they **enjoy** doing them. This is a trial and error process. They may have to try several things before they find one that suits them.

What have you learned?	
Write down 2 goals related to your rest and the baby steps it will take to reach these goals.	
Goal #1: Baby steps to reach goal #1: a) b) c)	Goal #2: Baby steps to reach goal #2: a) b) c)

Step 4: Balance

We have introduced many issues related to self-care. It may seem overwhelming (O.K., O.K., I am sure it seems a bit overwhelming). Not to worry!! This is all part of the **process.** The act of looking at how you treat yourself is a first huge step to a LIFETIME of positive changes. Just think about it, if you can develop a more respecting attitude toward yourself, since you are stuck with yourself for the rest of your life, the whole rest of your life stands to improve! Learning is part of this process. We take baby steps and learn with every step we take. Ultimately this is about balance. We are aiming to:

- Give some of your time to others but save time just for yourself.
- Balance what you have to do with what you like to do.
- Balance the amount you give to others with the amount you ask from others.
- Pay attention when things get out of balance and make necessary adjustments.

Don't forget the metaphor we started with: treating yourself as an honored guest.
To begin this lifelong process (that hopefully will start today), there are several

approaches you can take. Choose the one that best fits your style.

a) Develop two new daily rituals. Start and end each day by checking in with yourself regarding how you treated yourself on that day. Don't blame yourself for the day. Accept how the day went. Accept the choices you made. Tweak your approach, learn, and apply what you have learned to tomorrow. Ah, those key principles again.

b) Choose one of the goals you wrote regarding eating, rest, physical appearance, and balance each week. Work on one goal one step at a time.

c) Do you need to be more accountable? For some of you, the amount of goals may seem overwhelming and what is needed is a whole paradigm shift regarding how you treat yourself. (Often this is what your child needs). In this case, self-monitoring sheets like this one can remind you to check in on a number of areas so you can begin to treat yourself as the honored guest that you are.

My Daily Self-Care Guide

1. Check in with yourself first thing in the morning. Make a plan for the day.
   □ Done   □ Whoops. I forgot or avoided this.

2. PLAN time in your day to have a moment to yourself. Incidental time doesn't count. Planning is symbolically important. During this time, do something that you WANT to do. Read. Sit quietly. Nap. This is recharge-your-batteries time.
   □ Done   □ Whoops. I forgot or avoided this.

3. Set aside time for meals.
   □ Done   □ Whoops. I forgot or avoided this.

4. Establish a regular bedtime routine.
   □ Done   □ Whoops. I forgot or avoided this.

5. Say NO to something if you are out of balance.
   □ Done   □ Whoops. I forgot or avoided this.

6. Take a moment to look in the mirror and smile.
   □ Done   □ Whoops. I forgot or avoided this.

7. Consider something that did not go as well as you would like. Think about it. Figure out what to try differently the next time.
   □ Done   □ Whoops. I forgot or avoided this.

Balance: Learning to Relax

Over the years, I have encountered many parents (and children) who do not know how to relax or sit and enjoy the moment. Some of the people I work with are even afraid to be by themselves. This is not only terribly sad, but it is a very unsafe feeling. It means the person doesn't trust him or herself, and trust, as we know, is the basis of everything. Instead of despairing, however, we just need to learn how to relax! You can do it. It just takes practice. First, we need to use our process approach to focus on the moment we are relaxing rather than focusing on how much fun we should be having from that activity. Next, choose something to do. Doesn't matter what except it should be something that will expand your horizons or that you already know you enjoy (a new hobby, picking up an old hobby, etc.). Then do it. Just do it. Don't try to have fun. Don't try to get through it. Just do the activity and see what happens. Did you like it? Is it something you will try again? It is important to recognize that new hobbies will become more fun the more you "practice" them, so don't give it up after just one try. Give it several tries! Why go to all this trouble?? Well:

a.   It makes life more fun.
b.   It makes you more efficient in your work and other activities.
c.   It makes you more creative in life in general.
d.   It can decrease your stress and increase your lifespan.
e.   Why not?

Key Points

1.   Life is about learning and growing. If we just focus on the end of the road (THE OUTCOME) and don't enjoy and enrich our lives with the journey (THE PROCESS) then life passes us by.

2.   If you apply this philosophy to yourself, the end result is an accepting and tolerant attitude in which you strive to learn new things, pay attention to and respond to your needs, and enjoy your own company.

3.   If your child sees this change, he/she will have more faith in the advice you give as it seems to be working for you!

4.   When you start with self-care, the rest falls into place and you are prepared to deal with it when it doesn't!

5.   Examine the areas we talked about (hunger, rest, physical appearance, and balance) and take baby steps.

Weekly Goals

We start off easy. Your first goal is to ONLY FILL OUT #4 on your homework page. Yep, your only job this week is doing something nice for yourself

Questions and Answers

Q: This sounds great, but often I just have to work late and there is nothing I can do about it. Why do you focus so much on sleep?

A: Hmm. I am actually going to turn that one back on you. Why do you think I focus so much on sleep? Did you know that sleep deprivation is actually used cruelly as a form of psychological torture? That animals die when deprived of sleep? That our stress hormones are elevated when we don't sleep enough making the whole day more edgy? If you give your body enough sleep, your brain rewards you by learning and your body rewards you by being efficient.

Q: I believe in the importance of self-care and balance, but I just don't have time for it right now with all of the time that I am putting into my child's recovery. Which one would you rather I choose, self-care or caring for my child?

A: Well actually, it can't be a choice. If you don't take care of yourself during the journey of your child's illness, you will burn out quicker than a firefly with no air. Seriously, being effective in a time of stress takes a clear head. There is no way you can do this if you don't care for yourself along the way. I have seen too many people try and fail.

It is a challenge to make time for regular meals, sleep, relaxation and exercise during the best of circumstances; when your child is ill, it becomes an unbelievable challenge. Truly, though, there is no greater gift that you can give your child than modeling these things for them now. We don't want them to believe that being an adult means self-neglect. So if you're having a hard time justifying doing it for yourself right now, do it for them.

Q: My child is always asking me how she looks or whether it looks like she has gained weight. What should I say?

A: Ah, another excellent question. As we briefly mentioned earlier, usually when your child is asking questions about their appearance they are often on top of their own wave. Thus, this is no answer that you can give that will satisfy them other than "No, you look like you lost weight." Unfortunately, that answer doesn't help because although it may decrease their anxiety in the short term, it also gives fuel to their disorder. A better strategy is to have a conversation about these frequent requests for reassurance (not during a time when your child is asking for reassurance but in a calm moment) and asking why she keeps asking you about her appearance and does that help her to keep asking. There is actually research to show that such frequent checking and rechecking about appearance is not helpful at all – it just keeps the focus on the disorder. Instead, a much more effective strategy is to really work on your own body image and self-comfort. Then, your child can learn by example.

Wisdom of the Week: My Gift to Myself

Go ahead. Find a new hobby. You know you want to.

Date:

Remember our key guidelines
It's a process! Try, tweak, grow and learn.
Self-parenting: a necessary prerequisite for other parenting.
Learn how to SURF The WAVE!
Remain genuine.

Unhealthy or unhelpful behavior I will discuss WITH my child this week and our plan to address it.

Eats too little	Eats too little variety	Exercises too much
Throws up after meals	Doesn't get enough sleep	Doesn't set limits
Abuses laxatives	Engages in self-harm	Other

Possible Suggestions of How to Address:
☐ Ignore it
☐ Have a discussion about needed change in behavior
  (discuss a future, necessary, logical consequence
  given the severity of the behavior)
☐ Implement a logical consequence (reminding your
  child of the importance of health before anything)
☐ Appeal to your child's inner wisdom (have a discuss-
  ion with your child about what you have observed,
  why you are concerned, the change in behavior
  expected)
☐ Reverse Time-Out (you leave)
☐ Group Time-Out (everyone leaves for 10 minutes)
☐ Regrouping (family meeting to get out of power
  struggle)
☐ Humor

My Plan:

Would a discussion be a good idea?

Heathy Coping Strategy I will address with my child this week and my plan to address it.

Express negative emotions effectively	Ask for more help	Set more limits (cut down study time, set a regular bedtime, cut out an activity)
Express an opinion- even if someone may disagree	Be more considerate of others	Place more realistic demands on oneself (consider the cost, not whether the demands are achieved)
Get a better balance of work and leisure	View a situation with curiosity rather than with criticism	Manage disappointing results
Share a vulnerability with someone	Embrace and learn from mistakes rather than running from them	Resolve a conflict
Tune in and respond more to what your feelings are telling you	Take more pride in oneself (being a more respectful self-parent)	Strut
Be Silly or just take yourself less seriously	Smile at your reflection	Initiate plans
Try something new	Get Messy	Break a ritual
Get more sleep	Other	Other

Possible Suggestions:	**My Plan:**
☐ Positive attention when takes a step toward behavior ☐ One-on-one time outside of eating disorder stuff ☐ Earning a logical privilege given increased health ☐ Praise and STOP – no BUTS ☐ Role Model Behavior Yourself ☐ Open the door for a discussion ☐ Set a limit ☐ Offer to teach ☐ Other	

Heathy Coping Strategy I will Role Model this week.

Possible Suggestions:	**My Plan:**
☐ Delegate something. ☐ Say 'no' to some things. ☐ Be honest with my feelings. ☐ Express my feelings when not on the wave. ☐ Ask for help. ☐ Set healthy limits between my needs and those of others. ☐ Listen with full attention. ☐ Praise and STOP. ☐ Say "I'm sorry" with no excuses. ☐ Allow family members to make mistakes without jumping in. ☐ Be consistent. ☐ Address negative self-talk. ☐ Be reliable.	

Self-care Strategy I will implement this week

Possible Suggestions:	**My Plan:**
☐ Make regular mealtimes a priority. ☐ Set a regular bedtime. ☐ Learn a new hobby. ☐ Spend some time with my friends. ☐ Spend time ALONE with my spouse. ☐ Set a regular time I stop work each day. ☐ Take weekends off. ☐ Buy something for myself. ☐ Exercise in a MODERATE manner. ☐ Take pride in my physical appearance.	No lame excuses!!

TIP OF THE WEEK: Balance.

CHAPTER TEN: Creating a Healthy Meal Environment

Where You Are

✓ At this point, you have learned so much, it is too much to type!   So, let's stick with the fundamentals!

Whenever you feel overwhelmed, take a step back and remember our main messages.   They should help to direct you where you need to go.

Key Messages
It's a process: try, tweak, learn, grow.
"Self-parenting" is a necessary step for "other parenting."
Stay off the WAVE.
Remain genuine.

Topic: Building a team around mealtimes

Ahhhhhh......mealtimes. At about this time, I often hear parents complaining that they find no joy in eating. This may be because eating is associated with the eating disorder. The stress of managing the disorder may have carried over and affected your own attitude toward eating. Or, you may have always had some fears about eating yourself. Regardless, this section is devoted to improving the mealtime environment in your home and to helping you and your child deal with any fears you may have related to eating and weight regulation. Thus, we will address the ENTIRE meal environment. By entire, we mean both the physical and mental environment of mealtimes.

The first place to begin is with what you, as parents, are responsible for in regard to mealtimes in your home. We delineate four primary jobs that we are putting you in charge of. We'll go through each one in detail. Sit back. Relax. This section could change your entire outlook toward mealtimes.

Your Job:

* Establish structured mealtimes.
* Work to create a pleasant PHYSICAL meal environment.
* Take responsibility for your own behavior at mealtimes and don't contribute to an   "outcome-focused" mealtime environment.
* Facilitate the preparation of balanced, flexible meals that feature a variety of foods.
* Role model a joy in eating as well as flexible, healthy eating habits.

Our Enemy: The "typical" family meal – chaotic, haphazard, loud, disorganized.

FEAR NOT! We can triumph over this obstacle.

OUR MISSION: MAKE MEALTIMES SPECIAL.

Step One: Establish regular, predictable, mealtimes.

Why?

We actually take a strong stand on this issue. Family mealtimes are VERY important. They are important for many reasons. Yep. Sit back. You are about to hear them.

1) Children can't learn healthy eating habits from you if they don't see them role modeled by you. Mealtimes do this.

2) Children need to know that there is a time each day when they get to check in with their parents. It makes them feel special. Having regular mealtimes provides this time.

3) Research shows that children who have regular mealtimes with their family have more positive physical and mental health outcomes than those who don't.

4) Children do better with structure. Having a reliable structure to family life helps to decrease anxiety and helps a child to feel secure. Regular mealtimes are part of this structure.

5) Adolescence is a difficult time. When the family becomes like ships passing in the night, this can add to an adolescent's sense of loneliness. Mealtimes communicate that time together is important and that the adolescent herself is important.

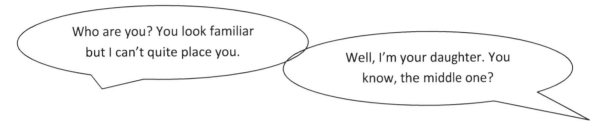

Who are you? You look familiar but I can't quite place you.

Well, I'm your daughter. You know, the middle one?

Well, although the problem in this scenario is obvious, the solution is a lot less so. This is actually the biggest barrier we have to contend with: the dreaded SCHEDULING PROBLEM. Before we problem solve some solutions, let's consider a few facts about adolescents.

Myth #1: My adolescent doesn't need me anymore, and I am badly stifling her social life by having her eat meals with the family.

Despite their whining, protests, complaints, insults, and fierce debates, your adolescent still needs and wants you to show that you care. It shows that mealtime with the family are more important than work, more important than extra-curricular activities. Remember, it's all about balance. Thus, getting past the schedule barrier and having regular mealtimes/family time is still very important. Even for an adolescent. I find that more often, children are jealous of their friend's families' mealtimes, if they have any reaction at all. However, if this is truly a concern, pick one night each week the children can invite a friend over for dinner.

Myth #2: If my child is not busy every second of the day, she will turn into a lazy sloth.

This belief seems to be a cultural disease. We could write a whole book on the development of this ideology, but we'll spare you that. Instead, suffice it to say that it's not true. We all need some down time AND we all need to be able to entertain ourselves. In short, we could all use a little more emphasis on being in the moment and a lot LESS emphasis on being BUSY, BUSY, BUSY; which brings us back to mealtimes. They are important. If they are not happening because of schedules, then we have a few choices:

Option #1: Some activities just have to go.

I have worked with many families in which the mere suggestion of this met with the same degree of enthusiasm as if I had asked them to walk barefoot on hot coals. Yet, as they made the changes and the family started to slow down and talk and listen more...well, you can imagine the positive changes.

Option #2: Be creative in the family mealtime.

If dinnertimes are truly impossible, then another mealtime may have to suffice. Perhaps a family breakfast or evening snack or afternoon snack would be a more reasonable starting place.

Bottom line: they need to happen. If they are not happening, then something else needs to go, but it isn't the mealtimes.

In the beginning...

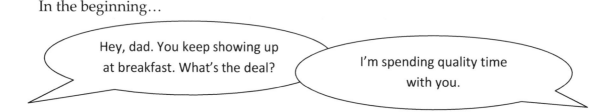

Tip Box
Trust & Expectations
Regular, predictable mealtimes attended by all family members do something you may not expect: they build trust. In particular, they build your child's trust in YOU. Why? Well, think about how we come to trust others. We can depend on them. They do what they say they are going to do. They are honest. Predictability and reliability happens when one of the rules of the family is that everyone comes to dinner and dinner is every night. You'll be amazed......

Like anything, having comfortable, joyful, and regular family mealtimes is a PROCESS. People get more comfortable with family time the more they do it. Making mealtimes happen is the first part of our equation. Our next mission to make sure these mealtimes are joyful experiences for all those involved. Intrigued? Read on.

Step Two: Take steps to make mealtimes more pleasant

As we have focused on throughout this program, in any situation, we need to take a step back and take control of those things that we have control over and learn to accept those that we don't. In the context of mealtimes, eating disorders can often take a huge toll. Parents come to dread them because of potential conflict. Children come to dread them because of potential conflict. Thus, inadvertently, we can bring tension to the meal via our body language and "karma" that negatively affects the atmosphere of the meal. How do we address this? Well, take charge of the aspects of the situation we have control over, and learn from the process.

We learn by association. If mealtimes are tense, conflictual, and chaotic, we associate them with stress. However, if we take steps to make mealtimes as positive as they can be, we minimize the negative impact of the disorder on these times. To do so, we may have to dispose of some MEALTIME BAGGAGE. If the thought of family meals is stressful, you are the victim of MEALTIME BAGGAGE.

Think about what aspect of mealtimes you associate with negativity. Your immediate answer is probably "the eating disorder" but it may go a lot farther than that. It may be that you have had your own struggles with weight management. Your family mealtimes growing up may not have been positive. Perhaps they were times of family conflict. Or perhaps you don't have many memories of family meals. We spend part of the next section addressing attitudes toward food and mealtimes. In this chapter, we are going to cast those attitudes briefly aside and focus on the PHYSICAL aspects of the meal environment.

The Physical Environment

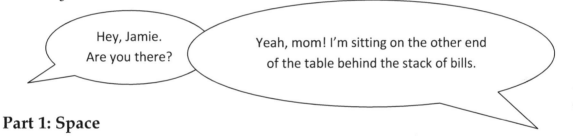

Part 1: Space

By physical space, we mean the physical environment in which your family eats their meal. The physical space and the tone of that space are VERY IMPORTANT. Our physical environment can either increase stress or help to create a sense of calm. If you don't believe me, go clean out your car. Really clean it. Notice how less stressed you feel as you get into it.

Are we saying that having a peaceful and calming eating environment will cure your child's eating disorder? Of course not. What we are saying is that subtle associations affect our mood and our stress level. While there are many things that are out of our control, we can take control of the peace and serenity of our eating environment. Will it help your child to eat? Well, it certainly can't hurt – and it might help all of you through this difficult process.

Think about the following factors as they relate to your own eating area. As always, we give some suggestions for each area, but only you know your family. Some suggestions may reflect your style, some may not. However, be careful before you rule something out without trying it. I have had very cynical parents come to fall in love with finding new candles for the table.

Clutter: Get it out of there!

- Clear the table.
- Get rid of stacks of stuff everyone in the kitchen.

Space: Make sure everyone has enough room to wiggle in their seats.

- Believe it or not, a lack of space creates stress.

Beauty: Beauty brings joy; joy brings calm; calm makes you stay off the wave.

Set a beautiful table. Don't do it alone. Your children need to feel important. Bringing beauty to the table (flowers, candles, nice place settings) is a great way for your children to feel like they are doing something to help with family teamwork. Go ahead, ask their advice. Make one of them in charge of the centerpiece and explore different craft projects to make some nifty ones. Let go of that perfectionism! This can be fun. Nothing like a gaudy centerpiece to lighten the mood a bit.

Part 2: Noise

Don't forget about noise pollution! Mealtimes should be QUIET. No TV. No video games. Want to experiment with calming music in the background, go for it – but heavy metal may be pushing things.

What's that annoying background noise?

Dear, that's actually your son trying to talk to you. You have become so used to sportscast announcers that I think you have forgotten what a child's voice sounds like.

Part 3: Smells

The smells arising from food cooking can be truly wonderful. Capitalize on this. Get creative. Maybe you and your children can learn new cooking skills: making homemade bagels. candies, etc. The smell alone may be worth it.

Tip Box
Trust & Expectations

- Assign family members different parts of the kitchen to keep free of clutter.
- Buy some organizational things to organize kitchen clutter (adolescents are master at tasks like this).
- Clear the table before every meal. Great job for someone!
- Give serious consideration to flowers or candles – beauty does help.
- Move around furniture. Nothing like a fresh start.

The Mental Environment

O.K. Now that you've made some changes so meals as a family can occur regularly, and you've thought about making the physical space more relaxing, we can move on to our next mission: examining the mental space of mealtimes. To bring back or maintain the joy of sharing a meal with those you love, we need to think about the "mental space" of mealtimes. A reminder is probably helpful here. Ultimately, you only control your own emotions at meals. Thus, this section is intended for you to take a step back and reflect upon your own mood and attitude as you enter the meal. If you take control of that time, you stand to most greatly impact the tone for the rest of the meal.

Insert a pause.

We rush around all day, working, running errands, driving the kids hither and thither, we rush home, slam something on the table for dinner, and gobble it up. Sound familiar? I frankly don't know how life got to be so QUICK. Given the emphasis of this program on learning by experience and being in the moment, I find it difficult to do much enjoying or experiencing if life is going by so quickly! Mealtime is the perfect example. Let's slow it down!

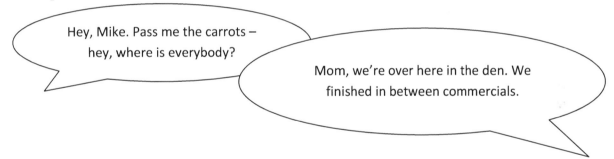

In order to make mealtimes relaxing, you might think about inserting a TRANSITION OR PAUSE. This is actually a tradition that I think has gotten lost. In earlier generations, it was not unusual for a before meal cocktail, mingling, a period of silence, or a blessing before eating; something of that nature. The point is that the family actually took a moment to stop and reflect before the meal officially began.

Think about your family. Maybe it is time to create some unique family traditions. In fact, this may be an excellent opportunity to get your children talking to older relatives. Have them do a little investigative reporting and learn about their grandparents' mealtimes when they were growing up.

Tip Box

- Begin with a word of thanks.
- Begin with a moment of silence.
- Have everybody stop and take a deep breath.
- Trade off telling a joke of the day.
- Have everyone share the stupidest thing they did today.
- Have a transition period. Allow a 20-minute easing into mealtime period in which you have fresh veggies or cheese and crackers out.
- Have the family come and mingle during this period. Then everyone sits down together.
- Bring back the before meal glass of wine with you and your spouse.
- Begin with a reading. Many religious traditions have a reading and response as part of the ritual surrounding a meal. Think about variations on this theme. Different family members can choose something they want to share.

Remember: It's a process! Baby steps. Try these things one night. See how it goes. Some of the more elaborate transitions may have to wait for weekends. Getting used to new routines takes practice. Don't throw out something new just because it feels a little weird, give it a fair shot.

Make mealtime protected mental space.

Remember, we form associations through experience. Thus, if mealtimes are when the family has their nightly argument or when the children feel put on the spot to report their grades, mealtimes will be anything BUT relaxing. We may do these things unintentionally. However, subtle messages carry a lot more weight than we may realize. Think if the following scenarios were a regular part of family mealtimes.

Outcome talk at mealtime.

So, how'd you do on that test?

Have you completed your college applications yet?

So, how much money did you make on that deal at work?

Feels like a board exam rather than a family dinner, doesn't it?

How about this? **Argumentative talk.**

This meal is terrible!

Why can't you get anything right?

What are you doing hanging out with those kids I warned you about?

Lovely, isn't it?

Instead, dinner times are vitally important opportunities to learn more about the other members of your family, to model critical thinking skills, you name it. How do you do it? Well, keep it PROCESS – ORIENTED! Ask about experiences and make it fun. Many families struggle with conversation. Thus, we are going to give you some conversation lessons.

Example of unhelpful questions:

What did you do in school today? Or even worse: How was school today?

Why are these unhelpful questions? Well, for several reasons. First, they are too BROAD. An entire day is way too much time to get one's mind around. It is exhausting to answer! In addition, it conveys a message that you don't realize. A broad question like that says "I don't really know enough about what is going on in your life to ask a specific question. Thus, I'll just ask you a general question because I am not really that interested." I know you are not intending to do this, but this is what broad questions do.

Examples of more helpful questions:

What happened today at lunch with Kara?

Why is this question a great question? Well, it shows you know enough about your child's life to know she eats with Kara, that you listened to what your daughter said yesterday and know that she and Kara just had a fight and that she was worried about seeing her today, and that you are interested enough that you will follow up and ask about it. A GREAT question.

Here are the basic tips for helpful questions:

1. Make them about manageable periods of time or specific events.
2. Make them about specific rather than general experiences.
3. Ask them to describe things rather than asking Yes or No questions.
4. Follow up on things you've asked previously.

Remember, this is about LEARNING. The more your family keeps talking at mealtimes, the easier it will become.

TIP BOX

Some things to think about when speaking to an adolescent...

Keep questions limited to a manageable time interval.

Asking about a day is overwhelming. Asking about a period is more manageable. Just think about yourself. Don't you get annoyed when someone asks "So how was work today?" I certainly do. Again, this is a PROCESS (can you say "broken record?"). Conversations get easier with time and you get better with practice. You'll see. The more you learn about your child, the more questions you'll have to ask and the more interesting and detailed the answers will be.

Don't be discouraged by monosyllabic responses.

Ah, am I familiar with the seemingly mute adolescent! My experiences have taught me that they probably did not start out that way. Rather, after years of telling stories which then results in: ADVICE, CRITICISM, INTERRUPTIONS, NOTHING...they have become silenced. You may have some work to do. You have to prove that you are a listener. You have probably made huge strides on this already.

Ask your child for advice.

This is a POWERFUL strategy. When you go to your child and ask their opinion, you are communicating many things – respect for their intellect, respect for their judgment, and respect for their wisdom. Boy this can make a person feel good!

Be willing to share about your life.

Even though they may pretend like they don't, our children are actually interested in what we do.

Open the door. Respect limits. Check to see if anyone is home every so often.

We don't always feel like talking. We have to be in the "mood". Thus, if you ask your child some questions and they clearly don't want to talk, leave it be, but exit gracefully. Something like, "Well, I would love to hear about your sessions when you feel like talking." Works like a charm.

TIP BOX
Experiential Questions

What did you do today in XX?

What do you think about such and so?

What did you guys talk about in such and so?

Listen to this thing that I read. What do you think about that?

What were your thoughts about that?

Did you agree with that?

Would you do something different next time?

What do you think I should do about such and so?

So, learn anything in such and so?

So listen to this…. What do you think I should do?

Did you read such and so? Why do think that happened? How could it have been avoided?

Want to make this more fun? Try buying the "UN-GAME" a game of fun questions designed to get a party started.

Chill Out.

Meals are only as enjoyable as the level of tension in the air. This tension can arise from a number of sources. We'll address a few. For starters, it may be helpful for your family to declare that mealtimes represent a truce. During this period of time, we put our anger and worries aside. Not only does this make the meal peaceful, but it is also great practice in emotion regulation! Does this mean you're being "fake" during meals if you are really and truly upset about something? Actually, NO. Effective emotion regulation is knowing that there is an appropriate time and place to express our feelings and a time when we are better off keeping them to ourselves. Mealtimes are peace times. Save it for later.

However, the truce is violated if you get anxious about the MEAL ITSELF. Timing a meal is HARD. If everything isn't done at the same time, who cares? Have the roast for dessert or put everything on the warm setting in the oven. Dinner running late? This may be a wonderful time to institute the before-meal cheese and crackers cocktail hour. New dish taste terrible? There's always a good peanut butter and jelly sandwich to save the day. People can make do, and you have learned that is a recipe that you won't attempt again.

You know something else that can really destroy a comfortable meal environment?? Negative or fearful attitudes towards food and eating behavior. This topic is so important that we have given it its own chapter.

Key Points

1   Family meals can be sacred, special times that create memories your child holds on to for the rest of her life. Make them a priority.

2   Many important things happen when family meals are regular that we don't realize: they build trust, they provide an opportunity for critical thinking, they allow your child to practice conversational skills.

3   The physical environment of mealtimes doesn't cure an eating disorder but can add to an overall positive aura around the meal.

4   The mental environment of mealtimes is crucial. Keep focused on experiences, not outcomes.

Weekly Goals

1)   Think about the eating disorder symptoms you are targeting. **Work WITH your child on choosing some common goals** if your child is able to contribute.

2)   Think about some skills your child needs to develop (asking for help or support, setting limits on self, etc.). Make some goals **WITH your child.** Think about some things **you** can role model in this section. Make some goals **for yourself.**

3)   Use these goals to create your homework sheet on the following pages.

Questions and Answers

Q: I couldn't agree with you more about the importance of family meals. However, I feel powerless. I am told that my child needs to be "well rounded" if he is to get into college. How can I risk my child's future by insisting on family meals?

A: I can understand why you are concerned. Thus, rather than reassure you, let's take a look at the facts. I have taken the liberty of copying the text from a highly competitive private academic institution in the Southeastern United States. Let's take a look at the type of student they are looking for.

"We want to find **the ambitious and the curious** students who want to tackle issues head-on and are **open to change**. XXX is a community of talented learners, and we look for people who have unique qualities, who can challenge us as much as we challenge them. **We want some bumps.** We want some students who are well-rounded, some with sharp edges. We want people who are not afraid to undertake things that are messy, complex, and extremely difficult to do well—because they love it. We like students who already know what it means to succeed and those who know what it means to reach and not succeed and reach again. **We like students who make intelligent and interesting mistakes, students who understand that only in risking failure do we become stronger, better, and smarter.**"

Do you see abundance of extracurricular activities written there? No. You don't. The emphasis is on values, integrity, critical thinking, and caring for others. They want students who explore the world with open eyes. These values are taught at the table. It is not the QUANITY of activities but the QUALITY. Help your child to become a critical consumer so they can explore the world around them with an educated eye and figure out the activities that are important to them and explore these to the fullest. Spreading oneself thin never works.

Wisdom of the Week: My Gift to Myself

Take out your social support inventory. I bet you haven't looked at it in a while! Reach out and touch somebody you haven't spoken to in a while. An email, a call, a card, whatever works!!

WAIT – A BONUS SECTION!

So what are some of the biggest barriers to establishing a happy and healthy meal environment? Oh the downright hassle of it all!

1. Hassle #1: Who's got the time? <u>**Hassle fixer:** organization.</u>

The more organized you are with mealtimes, the less time they take and the easier they become. First, think about all the stages of meal preparation. There is planning the meal, shopping, preparing the food, setting the table, and clean up. Delegate these tasks out. Make a set shopping day. Have a set grocery list. Make someone a salad maker, someone a potato peeler, someone a table setter; all these things make this a family process.

2. Hassle #2: What do I make? <u>**Hassle fixer:** develop a fun system.</u>

In the opinion of many meal organizers, the biggest pain is figuring out what to make. I have done many interviews and investigations to determine the strategies that different families use in planning meals. Here are their combined suggestions. Add your own (write me with them though so I can add them to the list).

1. Give each family member a night to plan.
2. Have a fish night, a casserole night, a chicken night, a beef night, a takeout night, a sandwich night, a breakfast night, an ethnic night.
3. Have a 'try a new recipe' night.
4. Get one of those 365 day cookbooks and have the cookbook tell you what to do.
5. Put all dishes the family likes on cards. Every Sunday pick seven cards to plan the week.
6. Feature a different ethnic cuisine every week. Mexican week, Asian week, etc.
7. Don't be proud. Convenience foods can save oodles of time.
8. Have a "make your own pizza', 'build your own baked potato', 'make your own wrap sandwich' etc. night; these can be fun and easy mealtime variations.
9. Create your own helpful system.

GOALS FOR WEEK #10

Date:

Remember our key guidelines
It's a process! Try, tweak, grow and learn.
Self-parenting: a necessary prerequisite for other parenting.
Learn how to SURF The WAVE!
Remain genuine.

Unhealthy or unhelpful behavior I will discuss WITH my child this week and our plan to address it.

Eats too little	Eats too little variety	Exercises too much
Throws up after meals	Doesn't get enough sleep	Doesn't set limits
Abuses laxatives	Engages in self-harm	Other

Possible Suggestions of How to Address:
- ☐ Ignore it
- ☐ Have a discussion about needed change in behavior *(discuss a future, necessary, logical consequence given the severity of the behavior)*
- ☐ Implement a logical consequence (reminding your child of the importance of health before anything)
- ☐ Appeal to your child's inner wisdom (have a discussion with your child about what you have observed, why you are concerned, the change in behavior expected)
- ☐ Reverse Time-Out (you leave)
- ☐ Group Time-Out (everyone leaves for 10 minutes)
- ☐ Regrouping (family meeting to get out of power struggle)
- ☐ Humor

My Plan:

Would a discussion be a good idea?

Heathy Coping Strategy I will address with my child this week and my plan to address it.

Express negative emotions effectively	Ask for more help	Set more limits (cut down study time, set a regular bedtime, cut out an activity)
Express an opinion- even if someone may disagree	Be more considerate of others	Place more realistic demands on oneself (consider the cost, not whether the demands are achieved)
Get a better balance of work and leisure	View a situation with curiosity rather than with criticism	Manage disappointing results
Share a vulnerability with someone	Embrace and learn from mistakes rather than running from them	Resolve a conflict
Tune in and respond more to what your feelings are telling you	Take more pride in oneself (being a more respectful self-parent)	Strut
Be Silly or just take yourself less seriously	Smile at your reflection	Initiate plans
Try something new	Get Messy	Break a ritual
Get more sleep	Other	Other

Possible Suggestions:	My Plan:
☐ Positive attention when takes a step toward behavior ☐ One-on-one time outside of eating disorder stuff ☐ Earning a logical privilege given increased health ☐ Praise and STOP – no BUTS ☐ Role Model Behavior Yourself ☐ Open the door for a discussion ☐ Set a limit ☐ Offer to teach ☐ Other	

Heathy Coping Strategy I will Role Model this week.

Possible Suggestions:	My Plan:
☐ Delegate something. ☐ Say 'no' to some things. ☐ Be honest with my feelings. ☐ Express my feelings when not on the wave. ☐ Ask for help. ☐ Set healthy limits between my needs and those of others. ☐ Listen with full attention. ☐ Praise and STOP. ☐ Say "I'm sorry" with no excuses. ☐ Allow family members to make mistakes without jumping in. ☐ Be consistent. ☐ Address negative self-talk. ☐ Be reliable.	

Self-care Strategy I will implement this week

Possible Suggestions:	My Plan:
☐ Make regular mealtimes a priority. ☐ Set a regular bedtime. ☐ Learn a new hobby. ☐ Spend some time with my friends. ☐ Spend time ALONE with my spouse. ☐ Set a regular time I stop work each day. ☐ Take weekends off. ☐ Buy something for myself. ☐ Exercise in a MODERATE manner. ☐ Take pride in my physical appearance.	

TIP OF THE WEEK: Add some beauty.

CHAPTER ELEVEN: The Joy of Eating

Where You Are

✓ You are now officially in the advanced chapters. Take a moment to stop and think about how far you have traveled. Think about what you do differently now. Think of all you have learned. Pat yourself on the back.

Whenever you feel overwhelmed, take a step back and remember our main messages.   They should help to direct you where you need to go.

Key Messages
It's a process: try, tweak, learn, grow.
"Self-parenting" is a necessary step for "other parenting."
Stay off the WAVE.
Remain genuine.

Topic: Meal Environment 2- Our Attitudes toward Food and Eating

In order for meals to be relaxing and enjoyable, we need to work on fostering a relaxed and comfortable attitude towards food and eating among all family members. So far, we have discussed the physical and mental environment at mealtimes. In this section we will explore our attitudes and beliefs towards eating and weight regulation, a source of great struggle for your child.

What does a healthy attitude toward eating and weight regulation look like? It's helpful to think in terms of balance. Healthy and relaxed eating requires balancing a number of dimensions:

You balance your hunger and your fullness. You try to eat when you are gently hungry and stop when you are satisfied.

What is balance? Well, balance is setting regular times to eat that you stick to (for the most part) like any other appointment.

What is a lack of balance? Waiting too long in between meals to eat and entering the meal starving. Eating too quickly and getting too full before you realize it. Eating until you are uncomfortable.

You balance eating for hunger with eating for random other reasons.

What is balance? Most of the time you eat because your body is telling you it is hungry. However, sometimes you eat because you are bored, the foods tastes really good, or you are at an event. We are all just human. It's when things like this become a pattern that eating like this becomes a problem.

What is lack of balance? Regularly using food for things other than our body's nourishment -such as eating for comfort, eating for boredom, eating to procrastinate, eating to self-sabotage, eating to hide from other things….ahh, we can use food for lots of unhealthy reasons.

You balance your attitude of self-discipline.

What is balance? Positive self-discipline involves setting limits in a kind and respectful way. We begin each meal with a mental attitude. That attitude can be: "Oh goody! This looks so good and I am hungry!" It could be "Oh, you can only eat such and so. Be careful not to eat such and so." It could be "Oh, I shouldn't eat that" or any of a ton of other options. Rather than coming into the meal with a pre-determined judgment, we really want you to think about eating a meal as a dance with yourself. What we mean is this. You prepare a lovely meal. You make yourself a reasonable plate of beautiful food. You take a bite. That is the first step of the dance. Your body responds. That is the second step. You take a bite…and so it goes. As you eat, check in with your body every so often and when your body tells you it is satisfied, then you stop eating. This is a pure and simple relationship with food -and an example of positive discipline.

What is lack of balance? Lack of balance is either negative discipline or no discipline. Negative discipline is: "You can't have that. Oh! You ate too much of that and now you can't have anything until tomorrow. I can't believe you ate that. How lazy are you?" In contrast, "no discipline" is "I don't care. Just have whatever you want."

Why is positive discipline the most effective strategy? Well, positive discipline is good "parenting" of yourself. It conveys "respectful limits." Fact is, we can't just eat whatever we want whenever we want it. We have to set some limits; however, unlike eating disordered limits, which are cruel, positive limits convey reason and respect.

It is important to understand this difference. When your child has an eating disorder, he or she most likely uses a "negative discipline" strategy. Sometimes, when they have embraced recovery, the relief of not having to listen to their disorder leads them to use a "no discipline" strategy. As parents, we are often so relieved to see this because we are just so happy they are eating. Indeed, this is often a normal part of the nourishment process. However, if this pattern continues we may need to help guide our children toward positive discipline. They are often afraid of this because they are afraid that any form of guidance resembles their eating disorder and they are often very afraid to go back there. Learning this key difference is very important for their sustained recovery.

You balance the time you devote to your eating with other activities not related to food.

There is a strange morality associated with eating nowadays. We seem to forget that we need to eat to live. There is nothing gluttonous about it. If we don't take time to eat and nourish our bodies, we will not survive. Paying less attention to food does not make one person more virtuous than someone who spends time and energy planning healthy meals. In fact, the people who put time and energy into planning and preparing healthy meals usually spend less time thinking about food than the people who devote too little time to meals. Huh? Well, the bottom line is that we CAN'T ignore meals. Our bodies won't let us. So, when people try to just "eat on the run" or skip meals, they often end up feeling more preoccupied with food and eating than if they just set aside regular time each day or week to plan and prepare meals.

What is balance? Balance is about setting time aside to plan and make healthy meals. However not so much time that this task greatly interferes with other activities.

What is lack of balance? Lack of balance is "eating on the run", not taking the time to plan to ensure your body gets enough food for the day, or spending so much time meal planning that you have limited time for other things.

A Self-Assessment

Stop and think for a moment about your history with eating. Do you have a joy for food?

A fear of food? Has your relationship with food changed since your child's illness, or have issues that you had already been struggling with come to center stage? Regardless of where you are, there is always room for improvement. Development of a healthy joy of eating will go a long way to promoting this attitude in other family members. If you have this attitude already, the next section will just be fine tuning. If you need to work on this, now is the time to pay close attention.

Getting back to pleasure. A pep talk.

Some people fear that if they were to admit that they enjoy eating and indulge this desire, then they would end up overeating. When I see this occur (repeatedly overeating a craved food), there is usually an internal war going on. The person loves the food, but feels badly about eating it. Thus, when a person like he eats a "forbidden food", he is not REALLY giving himself permission to have it. There is a part of him that thinks eating this food is really NOT O.K. Thus, in his mind, he may threaten to take the food away in the future. When he actually allows himself to eat, he may over-eat that food because of that potential threat. The way out of this trap is to truly understand balance. When we balance what our body needs with good reason and common sense, there is room for everything. We can eat a moderately sized portion because we know we haven't committed some terrible crime!

Tip Box: The French

French culture is a great example of why this principle does not result in gluttony but, instead, in balance and moderation. The French are known for their love and appreciation of fine cuisine. We're not talking low-fat cuisine either. Rich pastries, cream sauces, cheeses – these are all known to be parts of the French diet. Yet, despite ADVOCATING such delicious treats, the French have a much lower body mass index (a measure of weight for height) than Americans. In contrast, the philosophy of eating in the United States seems very all or nothing; we often view eating rich foods SINFUL and REPROACHABLE. Yet, when we offer them, we offer huge portions. What is going on here?

The lesson? If we get back to a joy of eating and a respect for our body, then we will eat a moderate amount of a variety of foods and we will maintain our weight. We will eat slowly, instead of "on the run" so we can pay attention to the messages of hunger and fullness our bodies are telling us. However, if we set up a rigid list of rules regarding food, think hunger is something to be ashamed of, and try to impose unreasonable standards on our eating, our plans will backfire and we will have a warlike relationship with food that may actually result in overeating.

Tip Box: The French…cont'd.

Instead, we could all use a bit more of Julia Child in us. For those of you not familiar with Julia Child, she is a famous chef who had a cooking show for several years on public television. Watching her work in that kitchen you felt her joy. You saw the beauty of food. Her joy of food and cooking (and of life!) is truly inspirational. We all need to laugh a little more in the kitchen.

Regular, predictable mealtimes attended by all family members do something you may not expect: they build trust. In particular, they build your child's trust in YOU. Why? Well, think about how we come to trust others. We can depend on them. They do what they say they are going to do. They are honest. Predictability and reliability happens when one of the rules of the family is that everyone comes to dinner and dinner is every night. You'll be amazed……

Bringing Joy Back to Food

Where do we begin? Well, it shouldn't surprise you that I have some suggestions.

STEP ONE. Use nostalgia to bring back positive associations with eating.

Think back to your early childhood. If you have a negative view of food and eating, try to think of a time prior to body image concerns, dieting, or other maladaptive views of food and weight. Imagine an event involving friends, family, tradition, and sharing. Was there a special food associated with this event? What was the significance of that food? What made it special? Describe the event.

Here's an example from my childhood to get you thinking.

> *My family is of Polish, German, and Russian descent, and these influences had a strong impact on the dishes prepared at family gatherings. One of my favorite dishes was an item called "sweet noodle kugel" a dish of egg noodles, cottage cheese, butter, eggs, sugar, and sometimes fruit (in this case, raisins). In addition to being delicious, this food had particular meaning because of the history it carried. My father and mother both grew up with this dish but both pronounced it totally differently. It was always interesting to me as a child to picture my parents as children in households that spoke "differently" and now who shared that experience. In addition, my father HATES raisins but my mom and sister and I LOVED them. To compromise, we would make half of the kugel without but my sister and I would try to be sneaky (well, bratty), and would try to hide individual raisins in to my Dad's half. Thus, kugel became a symbol of family sharing and fun as well as being a delicious treat!*

STEP TWO. Bring fun and beauty back into meal preparation.

What? Fun and meal preparation? Sound like an oxymoron? If meal planning and preparation are aversive experiences for you, there's hope. Narrow down what aspects of this process you don't enjoy. Oftentimes, our lack of enjoyment comes from a lack of time. In the Q and A section of this chapter, we offer some suggestions to make meal preparation more time-friendly. For now, we focus on the act of preparing the meal. This is where a positive attitude toward food can really be generated. THINK JULIA CHILD.

It is helpful in planning and preparing meals to think about your senses. Pick a sense that you really want to indulge. Here are some examples of how each sense can be awakened while you PREPARE the meal. Believe it or not, if eating disorders are forbidden in your kitchen (many parents I work with actually do not permit their child with an eating disorder to enter the kitchen prior to mealtimes because it makes the child, and the parent, so nervous), then this can actually be a relaxing time.

HEARING. We don't often think of the sound of cooking but you'd be amazed at the sounds you hear if you begin to pay attention. Think about the cracking of eggs, the whirring of a mix-master, the grating of the peeler as you peel vegetables. Notice the crunch of an apple as you eat it; use **Sound** to help choose your meals. Are you in a fun kind of mood? Make yourself a loud dinner. Crunch on water chestnuts, chomp on celery, brown some beef with onions – make sure everyone in the house knows you're taking over the kitchen. Slamming around pans is also a great way to discharge negative energy.

> **SOUND**
> For you music lovers out there, there are few things as energizing or relaxing as listening to your favorite music. Alone in the kitchen, listening to your favorite music and chopping away can really be a relaxing time.

> **TASTE**
> Don't let the eating disorder keep you from experimenting with new foods. Remember what we discussed in terms of balance. When you try a new dish, try to make some safe and familiar side dishes so everything balances out..

TASTE. Take the time to enhance the flavor of what you prepare. Think spices, think quality ingredients, think new dishes that you've never tried before. Watch a cooking show. Treat yourself to a few new cookbooks.

TOUCH. When we think about touch in relation to food we often think about texture. (Unless of course you have a toddler for whom touch means precisely that – i.e. how does the food feel in my hand as I toss it across the room)? Do you want something crunchy, mushy, firm, soft, etc. Ask yourself what you feel like.

SMELL. The writer Marcel Proust composed a literary masterpiece called Swann's Way in which he described how particular sensory experiences, notably smells, could carry us back in powerful, vivid ways to early memories. By recreating these smells and recalling these experiences, we can begin to reawaken a happy relationship with food – our love of food before it was corrupted by strict dietary rules and negative connotations.

SMELL

Don't let the eating disorder spoil a delicious smell. The family is a team, remember, and the eating disorder doesn't get to dictate what the house smells like. Some smells, because they smell so delicious, might scare the eating disorder because the eating disorder is afraid your child will be tempted to eat the food. How to deal with this? Talk about it. Delicious smelling food is nothing to fear. Promise that if your child feels "out of control" you would sit with him while he ate it. Whatever you both decide. What is not permitted is rude behavior. Thus, perhaps to protect themselves, individuals with eating disorders will often say something looks or smells "gross". **Call your child on this. No need for rudeness.**

Think of powerful smells for you. did the smell of particular dishes signify certain occasions? Symbolize family time? Get you out of bed in the morning? As you chose what to prepare, think about something that will make the house smell wonderful.

VISION. Use fresh, bright vegetables. Use cooking techniques such as steaming, stir frying, or blanching that maximize a food's color. Think about the vibrant orange of sweet potatoes, the lush red of fresh tomatoes and raspberries, how pretty a parfait glass with white creamy ricotta cheese, bananas and berries would look. Choose beautiful dishes. Set a lovely table with flowers. Remember all the meal environment aspects we talked about.

STEP THREE. Call a truce.

In order for you to be able to enjoy food and eating and to pass this attitude on to your children, you may have to call a truce, with yourself. For those of you who are struggling with your own attitudes toward food and eating, a truce is essential. I say a truce rather than a treaty because I know this is tough. It is hard to treat yourself differently and to trust your body if you never have. Think about trying.

Get back to YOUR BODY.

Well, in order to get back to using hunger to guide the amount of food you eat, you have to start listening. Makes sense, right? MANY, MANY, people have lost this ability, so don't get discouraged if this seems very hard at first. Two metaphors will help us here. Remember when you first learned to drive a car? It seemed AGONIZING!! You had to pay attention to every little foot move, hand move, checking the streets with hypervigilance, etc. It was hard to figure out how other people seemed to do this with such little effort. Then, as you got better, all these things became automatic and now you get to places and may not even remember the drive!

POINT: *If you are not good at listening to your body, it will seem to demand a lot of attention at first. It will get MUCH easier.*

Now think about playing darts. Your goal: hit the bullseye. You throw the dart. It is just right of center. Next time you throw you adjust your angle. Closer. Finally, you nail it. Fabulous! Learning to read your hunger signals is just like this. You learn to tweak the amount you eat in response to the different signals your body gives you. Over time, you will learn to adjust the amount you eat so that when you finish a meal you are comfortable and energized, not unsatisfied or overfull. The amazing thing is that once you and your body are moving as a symphony, your self-trust will increase TREMENDOUSLY. Where to begin? Well, we train many individuals in hunger awareness. Using a scale like the one below, we have them check in with their bodies before the meal begins, halfway through the meal, and when the meal is over. Over

Starving	Hungry	Neutral	Satisfied	Stuffed
(too hungry)	*(a gentle, stomach growl kind of hunger)*	*(not full, but not yet satisfied)*	*(Comfortably full)*	*(too full!!)*
1	2	3	4	5

time, their ability to sense these cues grows.

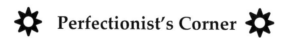 **Perfectionist's Corner**

Perfectionist: If I wasn't such a pig, I w2ould be able to listen to my body.

Voice of Reason: I strongly disagree, Mr. or Ms. Perfectionist! There are many, many factors that interfere with our ability to read our body's signals and not one of them has to do anything with a person's character. These cues become muffled due to our learning histories (e.g. being given food when we are upset); environmental influences (having food readily available); our mealtime relationship with OUR parents (having to clear your plate as a child); and many, many other reasons. Thus, you did not put yourself here, but we are counting on your to bring yourself out!

Steps of Hunger Awareness

1. Familiarize yourself with the stages of hunger and fullness in the scale above.

2. STOP whatever you are doing. Close your eyes. Take a slow, deep breath.

3. Take a few more breaths and make each one a little deeper and a little slower (we are trying to get you to clear your mind and focus).

4. Now focus on your stomach (for those who don't know, your stomach is about where the base of your rib cage sits. Some people confuse their lower intestines with their stomach. Although this is where the food is sent after it leaves your stomach, your intestines do not play a role in detecting when you are full or hungry).

5. Does your stomach feel like a 1? A 1 is when you are very, very hungry. You have not eaten for a while and you may feel weak or have a headache.

6. Careful to distinguish this from "anxious hunger" which is "I have to eat now!" We try to stay away from "1" because entering a meal too hungry makes it very hard to eat slowly and pay attention to your hunger signals.

7. Does your stomach feel like a 2? A 2 is when your stomach is gently growling, feels empty, and you feel hungry. We want to start eating here.

8. How about a 3? A 3 is when you feel neutral. You have eaten a good amount of food and you have taken the edge off of your hunger, but you are not yet satisfied.

9. Maybe you are a 4. A 4 is when you feel satisfied and you would feel uncomfortable if you ate anymore. About 20 minutes from this point, you will still feel satisfied but not uncomfortable.

10. Is your stomach feeling stuffed? Uncomfortable? Like you would have difficulty jogging or walking quickly? Then you are at a 5.

11. Think about where you are starting the meal. Stop halfway through the meal and give yourself another rating. Finally, give yourself a rating when you are finished. Consider this information gathering. You are going to goof up a lot. Sometimes you will overeat. Sometimes you will under-eat. However, the more you pay attention, the more skilled you will get at listening to your body.

Very Important Point: Hunger awareness is an advanced skill. Don't forget the stages of nutrition your child must pass through before he can get better at reading his body's signals. At first, because the disorder is so loud, it is much better to eat on a schedule, whether or not his body feels hungry. As he progresses and gets more comfortable reading his body's signals, the more we can trust his body's messages (usually this doesn't happen until he is at a healthy weight).

Tip Box: Getting Back to Your Body

1   Check in with your body throughout the meal.
2   Slow down. Put your fork down in between bites.
3   Eliminate distractions while you eat. It's hard to listen to your stomach in a sea of chaos. Thus, as you begin following the strategies we have described, listening to your body will get easier and easier.
4   Have a hot beverage during meals and take a sip in between bites.
5   Take a deep breath before you start eating and check in with yourself before you pick up the fork.
6   Avoid having a predetermined amount in your mind before you start to eat. Try to use your body as a guide instead.

Key Points.

1) Remember, little changes add up.
2) Look at your own attitudes towards food and eating.
3) Focus on reawakening a fun attitude towards food. There's a Julia Child in all of us!!
4) Get tuned into your own body. Use your hunger to guide your food choices.

Friendly reminders from Chapters 10 and 11

Be open to trying new foods.
There is no need to discuss the nutritional information of a meal.
No conflict at mealtimes.
Don't forget the mealtime truce. Insert a PAUSE.
Mealtimes are for listening not lectures.
Your children are watching you.
Feed your hunger.
Leave outcomes out of meals. In fact, leave them out outside of meals.

Questions and Answers

Q: My child is eating so much now. It is wonderful to see and is such a huge relief. However, she is eating so much that I am afraid she will become a binge eater or will put on weight too quickly and will have a relapse.

A: This happens very often when someone has been starving. Remember in the first section when we talked about how an eating disorder destroys an individual's trust in himself? Why? Well, in first section we discussed how we are all our own parents, and we must take care of our body's needs. In the case of an eating disorder, the individual is starving herself and neglecting these needs. A very scary situation, indeed. Several things happen when an individual with an eating disorder who has been starving herself starts to eat. First, her body has a tremendous amount of repair work to do. Thus, her body NEEDS a lot of food. Some individuals require as many as 5000 calories a day when their body starts to rebuild. Second, your child is both relieved and afraid at the same time. She is relieved that the family has joined together to help her fight this dangerous part of her. However, she is often afraid to go back to the state of extreme restriction and starvation. Thus, she may have a fear of exerting any limits on her eating. This is where our lesson of positive discipline comes in! We need to help our child learn gentle, loving limits.

How? Start with her pace of eating. Make sure she continues to eat slowly and teach her how to begin to check in with her body as you are "relearning." Warn her that this will take practice and that she will make mistakes just like you will. Help her to be patient with herself.

Wisdom of the Week: My Gift to Myself

Our wisdom of the week introduces us to an oral tradition called "lectio." The purpose of lectio is to derive a deep sense of meaning from the written word and to share this deeper meaning with others. Have you ever read a passage following which your immediate response was "I have to read this or share this with someone?" In essence, this reading has touched us in a deep way, and we wish to share that experience with others so that they may benefit from this special moment. Such is the essence of lectio (among many of the adolescents I work with, they describe this phenomenon in terms of music that they hear).

So what bearing does this have on mealtimes? Imagine if, one night a week, you were to start the meal off with a passage. Each member of the family would be given a night. On his night, that family member would read a brief passage to the family that was particularly meaningful to him. What a beautiful and special tradition that would be!

Such a ritual may not suit your family. However, I encourage you to open your minds to create unique family traditions that may bring back to mealtimes that sense of sacred sharing that has been lost for many families.

Date:

Remember our key guidelines

It's a process! Try, tweak, grow and learn.

Self-parenting: a necessary prerequisite for other parenting.

Learn how to SURF The WAVE!

Remain genuine.

Unhealthy or unhelpful behavior I will discuss WITH my child this week and our plan to address it.

Eats too little	Eats too little variety	Exercises too much
Throws up after meals	Doesn't get enough sleep	Doesn't set limits
Abuses laxatives	Engages in self-harm	Other

Possible Suggestions of How to Address:

☐ Ignore it

☐ Have a discussion about needed change in behavior
  (discuss a future, necessary, logical consequence given the severity of the behavior)

☐ Implement a logical consequence (reminding your child of the importance of health before anything)

☐ Appeal to your child's inner wisdom (have a discussion with your child about what you have observed, why you are concerned, the change in behavior expected)

☐ Reverse Time-Out (you leave)

☐ Group Time-Out (everyone leaves for 10 minutes)

☐ Regrouping (family meeting to get out of power struggle)

☐ Humor

My Plan:

Would a discussion be a good idea?

Heathy Coping Strategy I will address with my child this week and my plan to address it.

Express negative emotions effectively	Ask for more help	Set more limits (cut down study time, set a regular bedtime, cut out an activity)
Express an opinion- even if someone may disagree	Be more considerate of others	Place more realistic demands on oneself (consider the cost, not whether the demands are achieved)
Get a better balance of work and leisure	View a situation with curiosity rather than with criticism	Manage disappointing results
Share a vulnerability with someone	Embrace and learn from mistakes rather than running from them	Resolve a conflict
Tune in and respond more to what your feelings are telling you	Take more pride in oneself (being a more respectful self-parent)	Strut
Be Silly or just take yourself less seriously	Smile at your reflection	Initiate plans
Try something new	Get Messy	Break a ritual
Get more sleep	Other	Other

Possible Suggestions:	**My Plan:**
☐ Positive attention when takes a step toward behavior	
☐ One-on-one time outside of eating disorder stuff	
☐ Earning a logical privilege given increased health	
☐ Praise and STOP – no BUTS	
☐ Role Model Behavior Yourself	
☐ Open the door for a discussion	
☐ Set a limit	
☐ Offer to teach	
☐ Other	

Heathy Coping Strategy I will Role Model this week.

Possible Suggestions:	**My Plan:**
☐ Delegate something.	
☐ Say 'no' to some things.	
☐ Be honest with my feelings.	
☐ Express my feelings when not on the wave.	
☐ Ask for help.	
☐ Set healthy limits between my needs and those of others.	
☐ Listen with full attention.	
☐ Praise and STOP.	
☐ Say "I'm sorry" with no excuses.	
☐ Allow family members to make mistakes Without jumping in.	
☐ Be consistent.	
☐ Address negative self-talk.	
☐ Be reliable.	

Self-care Strategy I will implement this week

Possible Suggestions:	**My Plan:**
☐ Make regular mealtimes a priority.	
☐ Set a regular bedtime.	
☐ Learn a new hobby.	
☐ Spend some time with my friends.	
☐ Spend time ALONE with my spouse.	
☐ Set a regular time I stop work each day.	
☐ Take weekends off.	
☐ Buy something for myself.	
☐ Exercise in a MODERATE manner.	
☐ Take pride in my physical appearance.	No lame excuses!!

TIP OF THE WEEK: Ask about things that demand description.

CHAPTER TWELVE: Understanding Perfectionism

Where You Are

- ✓ You have learned more about the program.
- ✓ You have learned more about the stages of parenting and how eating disorders take your child off the path of healthy growth.
- ✓ You have learned about strategies of parenting and emotion regulation that can help you be more effective in your role.
- ✓ You have learned about healthy nutrition and how this gets confused by your child's disorder.
- ✓ You have learned about behavior and the factors that keep it going.
- ✓ You have learned about the barriers that get in the way of behavior change.
- ✓ You have been introduced to our experiential/process approach to life.
- ✓ You are working on treating yourself with respect so your child can understand what that looks like.
- ✓ You have worked to make family meals special, sacred times of sharing and connecting.

Do you feel really smart now?

Key Messages

It's a process: try, tweak, learn, grow.

"Self-parenting" is a necessary step for "other parenting."

Stay off the WAVE.

Remain genuine.

Topic: Perfectionism: Where It Came From

You may have wondered why we keep mentioning perfectionism throughout this workbook. It's time to tell you why. Importantly, research studies have shown that individuals who are high in perfectionism have a greater risk for developing an eating disorder than those lower in perfectionism. Of additional concern, studies have found that perfectionism in parents is associated with hopelessness and depression in their children and in themselves. Pretty important, huh!

As we learn more about perfectionism, we have come to understand that there is a big difference between "**perfectionism**" and "**striving for excellence**." Understanding this difference is very important for your own mental health and that of your children. As we will learn, striving for difficult goals can be a healthy and adaptive process. Perfectionists, however, take this striving and turn it into something quite threatening and negative. We hope we help you to understand this key difference. If you struggle with perfectionism, it is important that you understand one very important thing:

YOU GOT HERE FOR A GOOD REASON.
YOU DEVELOPED PERFECTIONISTIC TENDENCIES, IN PART,
BECAUSE IT HELPED YOU TO COPE.

Our job is to help you identify perfectionism in yourself so you can channel that energy in a positive and productive direction. To achieve these changes, we will follow several steps. First, we will try to better understand where perfectionism comes from. Next we will help you to differentiate harmful perfectionism from positive striving. We will teach you how to separate healthy from unhealthy goals and work on how you respond to mistakes. Finally, we will point out "perfectionistic traps" that get people into trouble. This is important because we need you to teach your children how to do this as well. As you know far too well, perfectionism maybe hurting him or her – badly. Prepare yourself to embrace mistakes.

Tip Box

1. You may have had a tendency to be perfectionistic for much of your life.
2. At some points in your life, it may have seemed that your perfectionism served you well.
3. Just because something worked (or was accidentally encouraged) at one point in your life doesn't mean: a) it is still working or b) a different strategy couldn't work better (and with a lot less suffering).
4. As life gets more complicated (i.e. as we become adolescents and adults) black and white rules just don't work anymore.

What is Perfectionism?

It is always good to start by defining our terms. We will use the definition used by experts in this field, Gordon Flett and Paul Hewitt.

> "Perfectionism is striving for flawlessness. Extreme perfectionists strive for flawlessness in all things."

Where does perfectionism come from?

Well, that's a complicated question. Researchers and clinicians know a few things. First, we know there is increasing evidence that people may be born with a tendency to be perfectionistic. However, like most traits we are born with, this trait interacts with your environment to express itself: strongly, weakly, or not at all. You certainly can't control whether you were born with this trait. However, you can control whether you channel this energy in a negative or a positive direction.

We are going to briefly present some models suggested by researchers in this field regarding how the environment may interact with your natural tendencies. These models are adapted from an excellent chapter written on this topic by Gordon Flett and Paul Hewitt. We are presenting these models because we think it is important for you to get a sense of where your perfectionism comes from (if you struggle with this) so you will understand yourself (AND NOT BLAME YOURSELF) for where you are or who you are.

Models of Perfectionism Development

Social Reinforcement Model

According to this model, people become perfectionists because they only receive positive feedback when their behavior is superior. This may happen when parents reward only the superior results of efforts and ignore or criticize average performance. The child may be led to believe that love is conditional based on his/her performance. Interestingly, research has shown that even when feedback is consistently positive, negative results can occur because the message conveyed is the same – the results of your efforts are important. Such feedback carries additional negative consequences when delivered in a critical manner.

We may accidentally do this when we fall into one of the most popular **perfectionism traps: the "YES, BUT" trap** (more about traps in the next chapter).

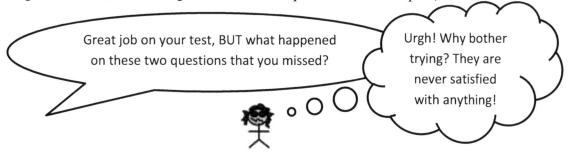

Social Learning Model

This model is perhaps the easiest to understand. According to this model, children become perfectionists because they see perfectionism role modeled by their parents. There are important things parents may **accidentally** role model that may promote an attitude of perfectionism rather than encouraging healthy achievement striving. Behaviors or attitudes parents may **accidentally model** include feeling shame, embarrassment, or guilt following a mistake rather than using the mistake as an opportunity for learning, refusing to acknowledge their own mistakes, or being so afraid of the occurrence of mistakes that parents don't allow others to try; and so many other subtle ways. We forget how subtle messages can have very strong meanings....

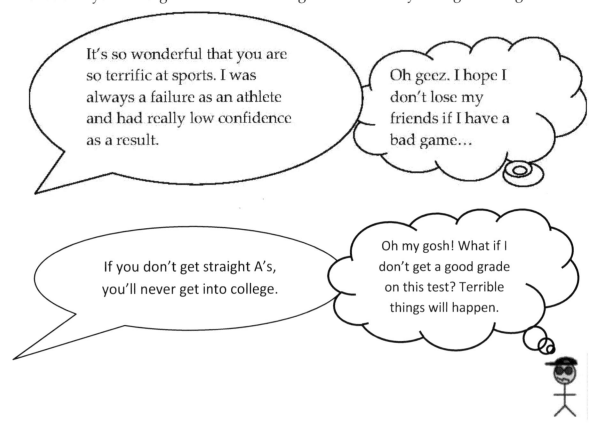

Anxious Parenting Model

According to this model, people become perfectionists because their parents often warn them about the negative consequences that will occur if their behavior is not perfect. Thus, task completion becomes associated with tension and anxiety and the focus is centered on avoiding error and punishment versus achieving positive goals. As we read about in the "PERFECTIONISM MYTHS" section, many of the fears that may drive this style of anxious parenting are not true.

✿ Perfectionist's Corner ✿

Perfectionist: O.K. Now you've taken things a bit too far.   I understand what you have said up to now, but the bottom line is, if you don't achieve a certain level of performance, then you won't be as successful.   Excellent grades are needed to get into excellent colleges and excellent colleges are needed to get excellent jobs. These are certainly the messages I seem to get from everywhere.

Voice of Reason: I can understand why you are struggling with this. There are many confusing messages out there. To a degree, "the letter" of what you are saying is true; however not "the spirit" of your belief. The problem lies in the emphasis and the extreme nature of the formula. If you emphasize the outcome, rather than the process (i.e. grades rather than learning), you may be creating a situation of such high anxiety that performance is actually impaired and joy is lost from the activity. By doing so, (focusing singularly on the outcome), healthy values are not being emphasized.

I am sure you feel it is learning that is important, right? If a child goes into a classroom with an eagerness to learn, the odds are very high that he or she will excel in that class. The worst case scenario is that he or she will learn a lot. However, if he or she goes into a class for the "A," she may just learn the material for the grade and not value the information and will often forget the material right after the test. Ironically, this emphasis will decrease the likelihood of getting a decent grade in the first place! Unfortunately, as a professor at a University, I have encountered this attitude far too many times. It is quite sad. People of good character, responsible values, with an eagerness to learn and a willingness to put effort into their work get good jobs. Period.

"Perfectionism is the enemy of creation."
John Updike

Social Reaction Model

According to this model, people become perfectionists because the rules they establish for themselves serve as coping strategies. Children need structure and limits. Structure and limits help children to feel safe and cared for. (This is often one of the hardest things for me to convince parents of.) Structure gives things a sense of normalcy and predictability that makes people feel safe.

The fact that people need such structure and limits is evidenced by the fact that in a chaotic or abusive home, a child will often create his/her own set of rules and guidelines for behavior. This structure may serve several functions. It may help her to feel safe and/or it may help her to attempt to avoid abuse in an abusive home. One problem is that children and young adolescents tend to think concretely. Thus the rules that they create are very concrete rules. Although these rules may work pretty well in the simple world of a child, when one tries to implement this rule system in an adult world, it is a set-up for failure as the world does not operate in black and white terms.

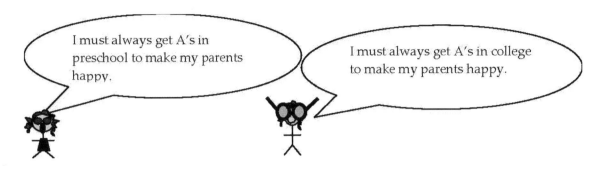

As you can see, perfectionism can come from a variety of places. If you struggle with perfectionism, it may be that a variety of these circumstances contributed to your current situation. Now let's move on to distinguish perfectionism from striving for excellence.

Separating the healthy from the unhealthy.

Many studies have been conducted that aimed to separate perfectionism from healthy achievement striving. This is just a summary of these findings. Basically, we will think of three parts to perfectionism: the goals an individual sets, a person's reaction to not meeting the goals, and the things a person believes will result if the goals are not met. Let's talk about each in turn.

THE GOALS

Research has repeatedly shown that setting goals is very healthy. Even setting difficult goals can be healthy. The goals themselves are usually not the problem. The problems usually occur regarding our attitude toward not meeting the goals. There are some exceptions, however, as some goals are just not healthy. Healthy goals have the following features:

1. They come from within. Healthy goals are YOUR goals. Set because there is something that YOU want to strive for and that is important to you.
Unhealthy goal: Going to medical school is very important to my father. I will aim to go to medical school.

2. They are not detrimental to health.
Following a goal should not interfere with your health, well-being, and basic self-care that we've worked so hard to achieve! If it does, it is not a healthy goal. Unhealthy goal: I must always study 4 hours a night even if I am tired, sick.....

3. They consider your personal strengths -at a given moment. Goals should reflect your personal dance.
Goals should consider YOU. We all have some things we do better than others. We also

have some things we are just not good at or don't enjoy. Our likes, dislikes, and strengths also change over time. Individuals are constantly changing. A goal that seems like a good idea at one time, may be a horrible goal at another time. The key here is flexibility and rhythm. This is yet another example of learning to dance with yourself. I used to want to cat. I hate cats now.

4. They are healthy enough to be followed by loved ones. This last criteria asks you to step back and take an honest look at the standard you have set for yourself. Would you be comfortable if your child followed in your footsteps? Hmmmm... not so cut and dry, is it?

Healthy Goals.....

1. come from within.
2. are not detrimental to health.
3. reflect your personal dance with yourself.
4. are healthy enough that you would feel comfortable if your children followed along.

How One Reacts to Setbacks

The second factor that distinguishes perfectionism from healthy striving is how one reacts when one does not achieve the goal one has set.

The Unhelpful

Someone who struggles with perfectionism reacts to failure with extreme self-criticism. He experiences the loss as a threat to his value as a person. He may feel very guilty for not having achieved the goal. After such a "self beating," trying to approach the situation again to try to achieve the goal is very difficult. Why? Well, think about the mental torture this person put himself through the last time he didn't achieve the goal. The thought of going through that again would make anyone hesitate to approach that situation again. As a result, perfectionists often struggle with procrastination – putting off approaching a task until the last possible minute. Because approaching a task has such potential for misery, no wonder it would be hard to start! Procrastination has one added benefit. Procrastination can be face-saving. It gives one a ready excuse if goals don't turn out exactly as one would wish.

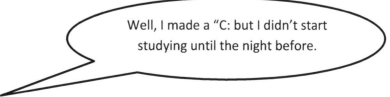

Well, I made a "C: but I didn't start studying until the night before.

Sadly, perfectionism has another negative consequence. Often it interferes with learning. Because mistakes are experienced as so painful, a perfectionist may struggle to acknowledge mistakes or may persist with a plan that isn't working in a desperate effort to make it work. Don't confuse this with persistence. There is an extremely important difference between persistence and inflexibility.

The Helpful

In contrast, someone who strives for excellence (i.e. "a professional") reacts to setbacks much differently. We're not saying he is excited about them – of course not! Sure, he is disappointed. Who likes it when things don't turn out the way one wishes? In fact, he may be downright upset. However, a "professional" has more of a process oriented approach to setbacks. Rather than just focusing on the goal, he uses the information from the loss as a way to take a step further towards the goal – or perhaps even to rethink the goal.

Thus, a failure to meet ones' goals is viewed as a learning opportunity and a chance to approach the goal again with this new added information acquired from the loss. Approaching the goal again is not threatening – it is but another opportunity to gain more information and to learn.

MISTAKES ARE OPPORTUNITIES TO GET WISER. NOTHING MORE, NOTHING LESS.

What One Fears Will Happen

Another important difference between healthy achievement striving/professionalism and perfectionism are the expectations a person has when a goal is not met. Perfectionists predict catastrophes or get so absorbed by not achieving the goal that they are unable to think of any alternatives. Professionals accept setbacks as part of the process. Common fears that I hear expressed by perfectionists are:

"People will think less of me if I don't achieve the goals that everyone expects of me."

"I will not be special if I don't continue to achieve in such a manner."

"If I don't do this well, I will never be able to do anything well."

"If I don't do this well, terrible things will happen."

Oh my gosh! I just got a "C: on this test! How can I possibly succeed if I can't keep up with my classmates! I'll never get into college. This mans I need to study 20 hours a day, 7 days a week.

Some of the people I have worked with describe the experience of a "brain freeze." When they don't meet their goal, they feel like a rat on a wheel that cannot get off. They can't stop thinking about the loss and all the bad things that will happen. Of course the problem with remaining on the wheel is that it makes it very hard to find a way out of the cage!

For those with healthy achievement striving, a goal is a step on the journey – to be reached for in different ways depending on where one is in one's course. Period. A disappointment is not a recipe for disaster. It is a disappointment – no more and no less.

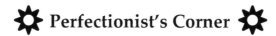

I am really disappointed by this "C". I am going to set up a meeting with my teacher to figure out what I missed to make sure I understand the material.

❂ Perfectionist's Corner ❂

A moment of reflection.

So why is perfectionism so unhealthy? Well, let's think about the effects of perfectionism on depression, anxiety, self-esteem, and most importantly, self-trust. Consider this:

Imagine you have a child. You speak to the child critically. You make unreasonable demands on the child without any consideration of the child's ability. You constantly warn the child of all the bad things that will happen if she does not do well. When the child succeeds and meets a standard, you cautiously praise her and warn her of the necessity of keeping that up or very bad things will happen. You fail to award approximations of success or steps towards the goal. Only complete success is acknowledged.

OUCH!! Sounds awful, doesn't it? Put a tape recorder in your brain for a day. You may be shocked at what you do to yourself. A similar tape recorder may be playing in the head of your child.

Given this, the following is not too surprising….

~ Perfectionism is associated with fear of trying new things since all new learning is usually associated with mistakes.

~ Perfectionism contributes to depression and hopelessness; in part, perhaps, because perfectionists never experience satisfaction.

~ Perfectionists have trouble approaching previous mistakes and learning different strategies since they fear the negative verbal barrage associated with another mistake.

~ Perfectionists don't experience self-trust. They do not dance with themselves. How can you trust yourself if you are never kind, compassionate, or considerate to yourself?

Perfectionism is toxic for very good reasons.

Perfectionism Myths

Before we move on and discuss how to address perfectionism, first let's take a look at some of the myths of perfectionism. These myths can sometimes serve as barriers to making positive changes. Thus, addressing them is important!

Myth #1: I have always been this way. I can't change.
Voice of Reason: I believe you. I think you have probably been this way for a while. I also think it has worked for you before. I don't think it is reasonable to ask you to change your personality. However, what I do think is possible, and infinitely helpful, is to get you to recognize your "perfectionistic tendencies", catch yourself in the act, and re-channel that energy in a more positive direction. We want you to think about being a **"PROFESSIONAL"** not a perfectionist.

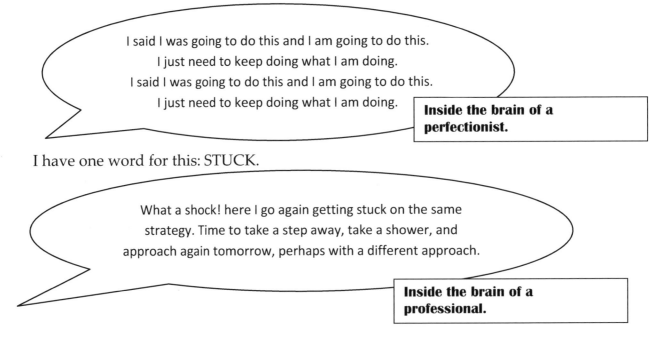

I said I was going to do this and I am going to do this.
I just need to keep doing what I am doing.
I said I was going to do this and I am going to do this.
I just need to keep doing what I am doing.

Inside the brain of a perfectionist.

I have one word for this: STUCK.

What a shock! here I go again getting stuck on the same strategy. Time to take a step away, take a shower, and approach again tomorrow, perhaps with a different approach.

Inside the brain of a professional.

Myth #2: Staying exclusively focused on one goal shows determination and extreme self-discipline. Changing one's strategy or goal shows a lack of willpower.
Voice of Reason: Setting goals and working toward these goals does show determination. However, incorporating feedback and learning from mistakes and modifying goals, if necessary, based on this feedback also shows determination – and wisdom. There is a difference between determination and stubbornness: between **perfectionism** and **professionalism.** Individuals with elevated levels of perfectionism,

sadly, often do not achieve the goals they set for themselves to the same degree as those without this burden. Instead, they get stuck in the same strategies.

What does a professional do, you ask? Well, it's time for a tip box.

> **Tip Box – A Professional...**
>
> 1 Picks herself up after a fall.
> 2 Accepts mistakes with dignity.
> 3 Is honorable in her motives for achievement.
> 4 Laughs at herself.
> 5 Rejoices in life, learning and sharing.

As we learn more about ourselves, we may find that goals that once suited us, no longer do. We may find that a former goal does not fit a changed situation. This is not about willpower. This is about life. Life is constantly changing and we, as humans, are constantly learning and growing. Wisdom and professionalism are about learning to remain steady in an ever-changing sea. The better our skills are as a captain, the better the ship shall float. Would a wise captain stay the course if an unknown boulder appeared? I certainly hope not!

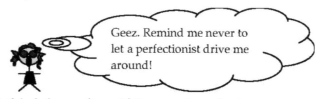

Geez. Remind me never to let a perfectionist drive me around!

Myth#3: People will think less of me if I am not perfect.
Voice of Reason: Many people I have worked with express this belief to me. They believe people expect perfection of them, would look at them negatively if they failed to perform, and sometimes provide examples from their past when people have expressed "disappointment" when they have not performed.

We need to take a step back for a moment and think about relationships, particularly quality relationships. Strong, healthy relationships are based on a bond of mutual respect and caring. People in a healthy relationship value the other person for who they ARE; i.e. all the abstract qualities (the quirks, the annoying habits, the idiosyncrasies, the characteristics, etc.) that make this person a person. If the strength or value of a relationship is dependent on the other's achievement status, this is a very unstable relationship, to say the least, as our achievement status is 1) constantly changing, and 2) different based on the vast array of factors that could constitute "achievement", thus what one person defines may different from what another person defines. Thus, for one person to be TRULY disappointed in another person because they are not "perfect" speaks to insecurities or confusing values in that person, it says nothing about your quality as a person.

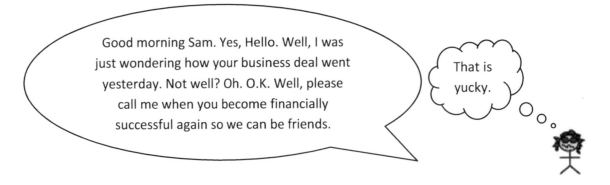

Ironically, acknowledging mistakes and flaws BRINGS PEOPLE CLOSER. Perfectionism actually DISTANCES people from others. This makes sense if you think about it. How do we get close to others? Well, one way to bring someone closer is via self-disclosure, revealing something about yourself that is private (e.g. a flaw, an embarrassing situation, something troubling you, etc.). Such disclosure makes your friend feel special because she knows you trust her. You have told her something about yourself that causes you some distress.

We all have quirks, flaws, weaknesses, annoying habits. All of us. It makes us human and it makes us special. When an individual refuses to admit flaws or to share them with others, it is very distancing. Why should we share our problems with people who "have no problems of their own?" Such individuals are not being genuine because we all have problems. Thus, sharing our flaws can actually increase a person's opinion of you because they know you are genuine.

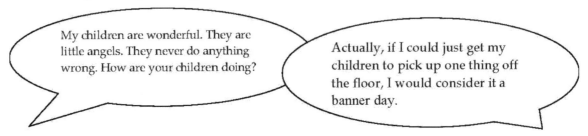

Who would you rather share with?

Myth #4: If I let go of this rigid perfectionism, I will achieve less.

Interestingly, there are two lines of research that demonstrate this myth is not true. When we place undue importance on an outcome and predict negative consequences will ensue if we fail to achieve the goal, our anxiety greatly increases. Although a little bit of anxiety can help us to get motivated, too much anxiety interferes with our ability to think clearly and actually impairs performance. This has been shown repeatedly in research and led to what is called the "Yerke-Dodson Curve." This is an upside down U-shaped curve that demonstrates the relationship between anxious arousal and performance. As demonstrated by this curve, a little anxiety can help to motivate us. For example, if you child didn't get "a little" worried about a test, he might not pull out the books. However, if your child (or you) gets TOO anxious, then that anxiety can get in the way of performance (and makes life pretty miserable!).

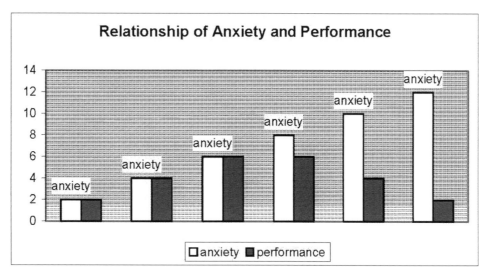

Here's another interesting study. At the beginning of a college semester, researchers had students fill out several questionnaires related to perfectionism and goal performance. They asked students to write down several **concrete goals** at the beginning of the year. Then, at the end of year, they repeated these measures. They found people who believed they "**had** to be perfect" compared to those that didn't, actually were **LESS likely to persevere** on their goals and had a **lower grade point average** at the end of the year!

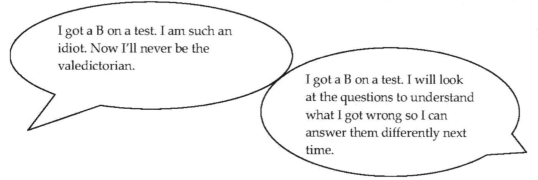

Hmmmm...I wonder who will be more likely to persevere in the face of difficulties.

Here's another interesting result from that study. They asked this same group where their goals came from. Did they form goals based on 1) What **THEY** thought they **SHOULD** do? 2) What **OTHERS** thought they **SHOULD** do? or 3) **THEIR OWN INTERESTS AND DESIRES**?

They looked at the relationship between the source of people's goals, the degree to which they kept working toward their goals (even in the face of obstacles), and the amount they achieved toward their goals. The results make sense. When people form goals based on their own interests and desires, rather than because they think that bad things will happen if they don't, they are more likely to persevere.

Think about this in terms of our process vs. outcome focus. When we have a balance between process and outcomes, we use the outcomes to guide our direction but are free to learn from each step along the way! If our focus is just on the endpoint, then we are constantly frustrated because the comparison of our current situation to our ideal rarely matches. It is hard to persevere in the face of continuous disappointment under these circumstances. **More on process-focused goals to follow.**

Myth #5. I will disappoint myself if I fail to achieve my goals.
People who believe in this myth may genuinely experience a barrage of negative self-talk following a perceived "failure." So, how does one deal with this flood of negativity? Well, let's think about **thoughts.**

Truth be told, there are few things in this world we control. Basically, we exert control over our own behavior. That just about sums it up. We can't even control our thoughts. In fact, the minute we try NOT to think of something, the more likely it is that we WILL think of it! Don't despair though, because we DO have some control in this situation. We control how we react to the thoughts we do have. We also control what we think about thoughts in general.

We control our:
1   opinion about the power of thoughts, whether we view them as random words that pass through our minds or powerful statements that convey the absolute, undisputable truth;
2   reactions in response to thoughts (whether we act on them or choose to accept them and watch them go by);
3   behavior; and
4   reactions to the thoughts and opinions of others.

Individuals who experience distress from their thoughts tend to view their thoughts as very powerful. They think because a certain thought or belief passes through their mind, it must be true and they must adhere to it. In contrast, individuals who view "thoughts as thoughts" can take a step back, keep their focus on their genuine goals and values, listen to the ones that seem useful, and ignore and distance themselves from the ones that are not helpful.

What am I trying to say? Basically this:
1) If you have always beaten yourself up for making a "mistake", then the next time you make "a mistake" insulting and/or guilty thoughts may pass through your mind, such thoughts are a habit, after all; however,
2) Just because these thoughts appear doesn't mean they are helpful, or true.
3) You have the power to decide what you do with them. You can let them cause you distress or you can treat them the same way we treat the eating disorder thoughts of your child – like an annoying knat that we just swat away! Thoughts are just thoughts, after all.

Tip Box: Coping with Thoughts

watch them go by.   Picture your annoying, insulting or worrisome thoughts as words passing through your mind. Watch them come in your left ear, pass through your forehead, and pass out through you right ear, wave them goodbye and greet them when they return to your left ear.

label them.   Hello, my insulting, demeaning thought. Where hhave you been? I haven't seen you in at least 20 seconds!

filter them for helpful information. See if they have any redeeming information to give, pull that information and learn from it, let the rest pass out of your right ear.

Imagine what Dr. Seuss would say about thoughts.....

A thought is a thought,
nothing more, nothing less.
I can't waste my energy on them,
Or I'll be in a mess!!!

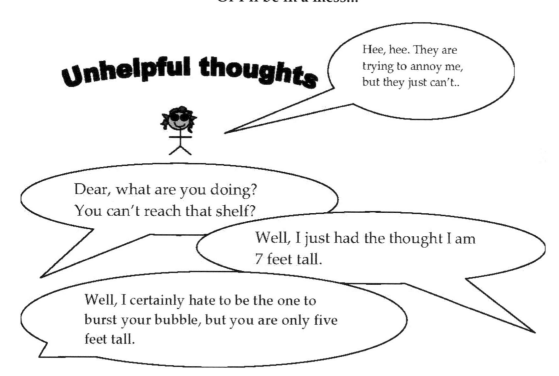

Yep, thoughts are random.

Myth #5: If my child does not succeed or is unhappy or…that is a sign of my failure as a parent.

Sit back. I like to get on top of my soap box for this one. Remember our discussion about control? Hopefully you do since we just talked about it! Well, in addition to not being able to control what we think, we also can't control others. That's right. We don't control the actions, thoughts, or feelings of others. We can do certain things, however. We can set up conditions to make certain situations more likely to happen, we can INFLUENCE others, and when our children are children, we have a fair amount of influence over the environment. However, there are certain things about our children that we can NEVER control. We can't control their feelings. We can't control their mistakes. In fact, trying to control either of these things is actually not helpful at all. When we try to "SAVE" our children from mistakes, we inadvertently give the message that MISTAKES ARE HORRIBLE. THAT'S A SET-UP FOR PERFECTIONISM!

Instead, we teach our children the skills to help THEM TO COPE with what happens. Parents can't save their children. They can teach their children skills and help them to use these skills. When their children have mastered the skills, they need to sit back and see if their children have learned how to use the skills. If they can't, we may stay back a bit and allow them to practice. However, if they are slipping badly, we step in and teach some more. Does this sound familiar? I hope so. You have heard this many, many, times already. This is the **DANCE OF PARENTHOOD.**

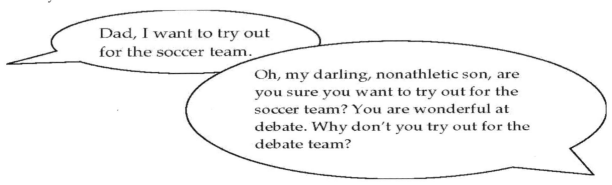

The untended message: If you are not a pro at something, don't bother.

Think about this. I am a psychologist. People come to me to feel better. If I had the power to make people feel a certain way, wouldn't I "cure" all my patients? Instead, I teach my patients skills so they can master their own emotions. My patients decide whether they will try to learn the skills and whether they will implement them. Thus, I am far from a "perfect" professional. All I can do is teach them skills and help them to clarify their goals so that they can make genuine decisions. The same logic applies to your children.

> **Tip Box**
>
> Approaching new, challenging tasks can be viewed as a scary situation or as an exciting challenge. Trying new things involves making mistakes. However, making those mistakes will help us to master these new tasks. When we pursue goals that are intrinsically valuable to us, we are more likely to pursue in the face of these obstacles. If try to protect our children from mistakes, we may accidentally prevent them from pursuing goals that are intrinsically valuable to them.

Myth #6. If you want something done perfectly, you have to do it yourself.

Well, that one is true. Next, KIDDING! For those of us who have been raised by perfectionistic parents, we may have picked up an unfortunate lesson. That lesson is this: "I want things done just so. It is easier to just do it myself to get things exactly the way I want them. SOOOO, I'll just do things myself." This may be true. It does take time to teach others to do things. In the moment, it IS easier to just do it yourself. However, when you do this, several unfortunate things happen.

1. **Your child doesn't learn how to do whatever it is you are picky about.**

Teaching your child takes time, but it is well worth it. Just remember, when you first started doing this task, you didn't do it very well either. In fact, you may have never gotten the opportunity to learn if your parent never let you.....This brings us to point number 2.

2. **Your child feels like you don't trust her or her level of competence.**

By doing everything yourself, your child inadvertently gets the message that he is not competent. We certainly don't want this as it may undermine our child's sense of self-worth! We certainly don't MEAN to give this message, but unfortunately, we are.

> **Tip Box**
>
> Teaching your children how to do things that are more easily done yourself takes time, patience, and a willingness to deal with an "imperfect" job. However, doing this is well worth it as it results in your child learning the task and learning that things don't have to be done perfectly to be O.K.

Key Points.

1   Perfectionism is unhealthy and unhelpful. It may also have worked for you in the past, although at great expense. Let's work to channel your perfectionism into professionalism so we can achieve without suffering.

2   Setting goals for ourselves is yet another example of the "dance with ourselves" we have been working on throughout this program. Healthy goals are sensitive to our shifts in movement. They go where we go; they don't stay rigidly fixed to the floor.

3   Let's take away the fear from mistakes. Mistakes are opportunities for learning. It would be terribly sad if mistakes were sources of shame or embarrassment.

4   Let's remember to keep our values regarding others as based on their genuine qualities rather than their daily, fluctuating achievements.

Weekly Goals

Laugh at your mistakes and take ownership of them.

Questions and Answers.

Q: How should I handle it when I am trying so hard to be a "professional" but everyone else around me is bragging about their children's achievements?
A: That is frustrating, isn't it? I have found, however, that the climate of conversations is exceedingly easy to change. Doing so has the benefit of helping your friend to broaden her perspective about her own values. Consider this conversation as an example.

Perfectionist: I am so proud of my daughter. She got the highest grade in her class again in science. How did your daughter do?

You, the Professional: You know, I have really been working to change my focus to my daughter's learning rather than her grade. The focus on grades was really putting so much pressure on her and interfering with her joy of learning. She had a marvelous semester in science and learned a great deal from that class and really enjoyed it.
It will take some work in the beginning, but you'll be surprised at how easily others follow along.

Q: What do I do about MY parents? They have reinforced perfectionism all my life.
A: Well, perhaps a good place to start would be to have them read these chapters as well. Just like you, your parents did the best they could with what they knew. You may be surprised at how willing they are to learn if it means helping their grandchildren. Remember, you can't control them. You can only set up conditions that facilitate their learning....

Wisdom of the Week: My Gift to Myself

Has there been something you have been afraid to try because of the fear of making a mistake? Maybe now is the time to try.

Date:

Remember our key guidelines

It's a process! Try, tweak, grow and learn.

Self-parenting: a necessary prerequisite for other parenting.

Learn how to SURF The WAVE!

Remain genuine.

Unhealthy or unhelpful behavior I will discuss WITH my child this week and our plan to address it.

Eats too little	Eats too little variety	Exercises too much
Throws up after meals	Doesn't get enough sleep	Doesn't set limits
Abuses laxatives	Engages in self-harm	Other

Possible Suggestions of How to Address:

☐ Ignore it

☐ Have a discussion about needed change in behavior
   (discuss a future, necessary, logical consequence given the severity of the behavior)

☐ Implement a logical consequence (reminding your child of the importance of health before anything)

☐ Appeal to your child's inner wisdom (have a discussion with your child about what you have observed, why you are concerned, the change in behavior expected)

☐ Reverse Time-Out (you leave)

☐ Group Time-Out (everyone leaves for 10 minutes)

☐ Regrouping (family meeting to get out of power struggle)

☐ Humor

My Plan:

Would a discussion be a good idea?

Heathy Coping Strategy I will address with my child this week and my plan to address it.

Express negative emotions effectively	Ask for more help	Set more limits (cut down study time, set a regular bedtime, cut out an activity)
Express an opinion- even if someone may disagree	Be more considerate of others	Place more realistic demands on oneself (consider the cost, not whether the demands are achieved)
Get a better balance of work and leisure	View a situation with curiosity rather than with criticism	Manage disappointing results
Share a vulnerability with someone	Embrace and learn from mistakes rather than running from them	Resolve a conflict
Tune in and respond more to what your feelings are telling you	Take more pride in oneself (being a more respectful self-parent)	Strut
Be Silly or just take yourself less seriously	Smile at your reflection	Initiate plans
Try something new	Get Messy	Break a ritual
Get more sleep	Other	Other

Possible Suggestions:	**My Plan:**
☐ Positive attention when takes a step toward behavior	
☐ One-on-one time outside of eating disorder stuff	
☐ Earning a logical privilege given increased health	
☐ Praise and STOP – no BUTS	
☐ Role Model Behavior Yourself	
☐ Open the door for a discussion	
☐ Set a limit	
☐ Offer to teach	
☐ Other	

Heathy Coping Strategy I will Role Model this week.

Possible Suggestions:	**My Plan:**
☐ Delegate something.	
☐ Say 'no' to some things.	
☐ Be honest with my feelings.	
☐ Express my feelings when not on the wave.	
☐ Ask for help.	
☐ Set healthy limits between my needs and those of others.	
☐ Listen with full attention.	
☐ Praise and STOP.	
☐ Say "I'm sorry" with no excuses.	
☐ Allow family members to make mistakes without jumping in.	
☐ Be consistent.	
☐ Address negative self-talk.	
☐ Be reliable.	

Self-care Strategy I will implement this week

Possible Suggestions:	**My Plan:**
☐ Make regular mealtimes a priority.	
☐ Set a regular bedtime.	
☐ Learn a new hobby.	
☐ Spend some time with my friends.	
☐ Spend time ALONE with my spouse.	
☐ Set a regular time I stop work each day.	
☐ Take weekends off.	
☐ Buy something for myself.	
☐ Exercise in a MODERATE manner.	
☐ Take pride in my physical appearance.	No lame excuses!!

TIP OF THE WEEK: Fall with grace. Pick yourself up with dignity.

CHAPTER THIRTEEN: Rechanneling Perfectionism

Where You Are

- ✓ You have learned more about the program.
- ✓ You have learned more about the stages of parenting and how eating disorders take your child off the path of healthy growth.
- ✓ You have learned about strategies of parenting and emotion regulation that can help you be more effective in your role.
- ✓ You have learned about healthy nutrition and how this gets confused by your child's disorder.
- ✓ You have learned about behavior and the factors that keep it going.
- ✓ You have learned about the barriers that get in the way of behavior change.
- ✓ You have been introduced to our experiential/process approach to life.
- ✓ You are working on treating yourself with respect so your child can understand what that looks like.
- ✓ You have worked to make family meals special, sacred times of sharing and connecting.
- ✓ You have learned the difference between perfectionism and professionalism.

Ready to learn what to do about perfectionism?

Key Messages

It's a process: try, tweak, learn, grow.

"Self-parenting" is a necessary step for "other parenting."

Stay off the WAVE.

Remain genuine.

Taking Steps to Help Yourself and Your Children

Regardless of whether you struggle with perfectionism yourself, one thing is highly likely: your child may struggle, at least when it comes to personal appearance. Our goal in this Chapter is to teach you strategies to help your child avoid the harms of perfectionism and re-channel perfectionistic energy into professionalism. We will start off by revisiting our process vs. outcome way of thinking. Next, we will spend a little time on our expectations – for ourselves and others. Finally, I will introduce you to subtle perfectionism "traps."

Step One: Focus on process vs. outcome

It should encourage you to know that we have actually been developing an "anti-perfectionism" approach throughout this program. How? Well, our emphasis on process vs. outcome is certainly a way to get away from perfectionism – a sole focus on the outcome – and emphasize what is important: living, learning, and striving for goals. We have applied this philosophy to your attitude toward yourself. We have applied this philosophy to family meals. Now we incorporate this philosophy more generally to how we run our lives. We will also practice this philosophy in two specific areas that are very relevant to perfectionism: the goals we set and the way in which we handle mistakes.

Tip Box: The Process of Change

Hopefully, with repeated practice, a "process" approach to life is making more sense. Just remember: this is a "process" -pun intended. Changing one's view of the world takes baby steps – and time. First, you become aware of how outcome focused your way of thinking may have been. Next you practice viewing the world a little differently. However, this "new" outlook just doesn't feel right because it is not comfortable or familiar. Like a new pair of shoes that are much better for your back, and keep out the rain, but geez, those old ones were so comfy…. But…….if you keep it up, gradually "process" starts to make sense, the pieces come together, you notice the tension going down, you start lightening up regarding things that used to bother you, you feel less threatened by new things……..It does work if you stick with it. And it gets easier.

Review: Process Vs. Outcome

If life is a journey, then an outcome focused approach views the destination as the only important part of the journey.

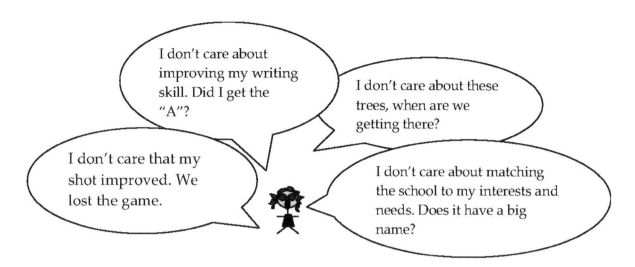

But what does a process approach look like in practice? How is it different? Let's look at some examples and then we'll explain.

Situation: You are having an emotional discussion with an important person in your life. **Outcome:** You are not honest about your true thoughts and feelings because you are too worried about the outcome of the conversation. Will this person be mad at you? Will this person think you are stupid?

Process: You are present in the conversation and use what the person says to figure out what you say next. You are comfortable knowing that it is OK not to have an answer to everything right then, but you can always request time to think things through. You are honest about how you are feeling in that moment and trust that if the conversation does not turn out as well as you wanted, you can have another talk to further increase understanding.

Situation: You are invited by a friend to take a class with her regarding a subject with which you are unfamiliar.

Outcome: You may refuse to take the class because you know you are not very good in this topic, may get a poor grade, or may appear foolish in front of the class.

Process: You consider whether the topic interests you and whether you would like to learn more about it. If you are interested, you take the class and are excited to learn new things.

Situation: You go to the gym to try your new exercise routine.

Outcome: You focus on the number of calories you burn, the number of minutes you exercise, etc.

Process: You enjoy the way your body feels as you get stronger, the feeling of pounding out all your daily hassles.

Situation: You go clothes shopping.

Outcome: You go shopping with a mindset of what size you should be and what size you are working towards and focus on the discrepancy between your current size and what you would like to be.

Process: You focus on your current size and your favorite attributes and buy things that maximize your current strengths and that you feel good about wearing.

Situation: You are eating out with friends and the people you are with are eating less than you.

Outcome: You think about the amount you "should eat" and make a rule about the amount you "should" consume based on what your friends are eating.

Process: You pay attention to hunger cues and eat to satisfaction realizing that the amount of food that others consume is irrelevant in determining how hungry you are at a given moment.

Situation: You are preparing a meal for company.

Outcome: You are extremely agitated because you are worrying about everything not being finished at the same time and turning out badly.

Process: You enjoy the process of cooking, play music, and have a lovely afternoon by yourself in the kitchen.

Situation: You see a very cute, thin person walk by.

Outcome: You berate yourself for not looking like that and ruminate over past choices you have made that have made a healthy lifestyle difficult.

Process: You realize the futility of comparisons as you know that everyone is a unique combination of personal history, genetic endowment, personality, life challenges, etc. and focus instead on what makes you YOU.

Situation: Your child is angry with you regarding something you did.

Outcome: You feel incredibly guilty because you feel that an ideal parent would not make her children upset.

Process: You realize that conflict is a part of all relationships. You listen to the feedback from your child and determine whether you need to do things differently next time or whether you need to help your child to accept limits.

What are some situations that cause you distress? What is the outcome vs. process ways of focusing on these situations?

Is this starting to make sense?

> **Tip Box**
>
> Process is viewing ourselves as a constant "work in progress", always striving to learn more about ourselves and willing to further develop our skills. We approach these tasks with an attitude of excitement and exploration, not guilt or shame.

To help our children with perfectionism, let's think about applying this process mindset as a WAY OF LIFE. The more you do so, the more it will make sense. However, in the case of perfectionism, there are two areas that are particularly important. These areas are: the way we handle mistakes and the way in which we set goals. Think about these differences.

Step Two: Apply Your Process Approach to Mistakes

Situation: You make a mistake and receive feedback from someone that you did something to upset them.

Outcome: You feel incredibly guilty. You feel that this reflects badly on you as a person. You defend the mistake because the mere thought of making a mistake is overwhelming. You beat yourself up, resolving to work harder and longer so this never happens again.

Process: You remember that there is no right or wrong. There are just experiences and learning. We try something. We get feedback. We see how it works. We tweak it. We go at it again. Each step guides us further along the path and helps us to determine if we have chosen the path that most suits us. With this framework, mistakes are not threatening, but just data to be used to learn something new.

Let's see what these differences look like in practice.

You know, when you gave that presentation, the graph was hard to understand.

| Innocent Feedback Provider | Outcome Focused Person |

Well, you probably don't know a lot about this topic. I am sure most people were able to follow along.

The result: No learning and no growth.

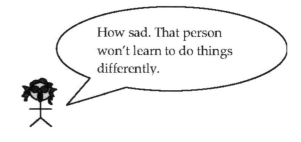

How sad. That person won't learn to do things differently.

How could the process be different?

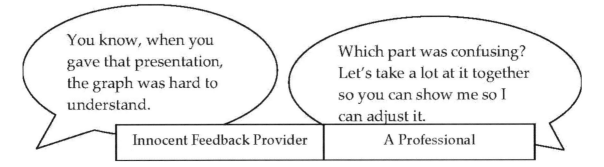

The result: Learning and growth.

Steps to a process approach to mistakes.

1. Look at the way you provide feedback to yourself.

Good feedback gives you somewhere to go. A next step. A way to learn. There is no goal to "outcome oriented" feedback other than to cut you down and make you feel bad. I have actually had some of my patients say that they are afraid that if they were to start being kind to themselves when they make mistakes, they are giving themselves permission to make more mistakes. Think about the research. This is not true. When mistakes aren't threatening, going back and trying again is MUCH EASIER.

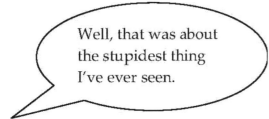

Great. That was certainly helpful. How exactly are you supposed to use this to help yourself learn?

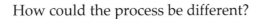

See? A next step here is clear. In which scenario is the person more likely to have found a solution to the problem?

2. Practice giving yourself helpful feedback. OUT LOUD.

That's right. Out loud. You need to become aware of how you treat yourself regarding mistakes. Your child needs to SEE AND HEAR how you handle mistakes.

3. Laugh at yourself.

One key to embracing ourselves as a permanent work in progress is our ability to laugh at all the misguided things we do and annoying quirks we have. Laughter conveys self-acceptance. It conveys we are COMFORTABLE with ourselves as a permanent work in progress. Try it. You might like it.

Tip Box: Laughter and Acceptance

Not only does laughter help us to accept ourselves, but laughter may also improve our closeness with others. Embracing personal flaws conveys comfort and confidence, and these qualities are exceedingly attractive. Think of Lucille Ball's sitcom "I Love Lucy." She was endearing as a character because she messed up all the time and just seemed to roll with it. We did love her – for very good reasons. One word of caution: laughter as a form of acceptance is very different than belittling laughter. We are laughing with ourselves, not AT ourselves.

---

4. Accept feedback with dignity.

Learning from mistakes also involves receiving feedback from others and being comfortable with the fact that we all misstep. Dignity involves listening to the opinion of others without defensiveness, validating the part they say which is true or possible, and giving their feedback serious consideration in thinking about how we approach this situation next time. This is particularly difficult to do when the feedback is not given with dignity. However, a professional remains professional even among less skillful behavior.

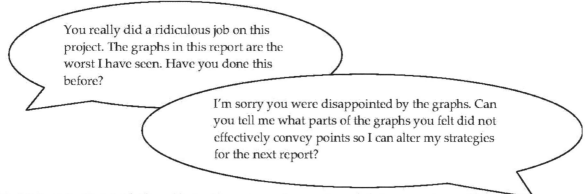

You really did a ridiculous job on this project. The graphs in this report are the worst I have seen. Have you done this before?

I'm sorry you were disappointed by the graphs. Can you tell me what parts of the graphs you felt did not effectively convey points so I can alter my strategies for the next report?

Huh? Is this dignity? Shouldn't this person have given his boss a piece of his mind as his boss was clearly rude in providing feedback? Think back to the emotional wave. His boss was clearly at the top of his wave and thus wasn't in a place to listen to logic or reason. Instead, this person validated the part of what his boss said that was true: his graphs could use improvement (all graphs can, after all) and turned the situation back to his boss so his boss then had to substantiate his exaggerated claims.

Applying our philosophy to goals

The second area we mentioned applies this process approach to the goals that we set for ourselves and the goals we help our children to set for themselves. To appreciate this section, we need to review what we learned in Chapter 3, when you learned how to treat yourself as an honored guest. This is important because in order to be able to set healthy goals for yourself, you have to have a good working relationship with yourself to start with.

A Good Working Relationship

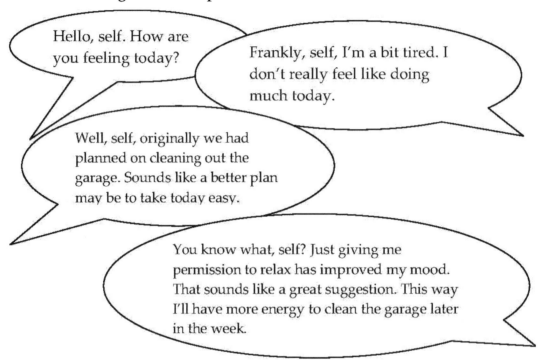

Hello, self. How are you feeling today?

Frankly, self, I'm a bit tired. I don't really feel like doing much today.

Well, self, originally we had planned on cleaning out the garage. Sounds like a better plan may be to take today easy.

You know what, self? Just giving me permission to relax has improved my mood. That sounds like a great suggestion. This way I'll have more energy to clean the garage later in the week.

Tip Box: General Guidelines of a Process-Based Focus toward Ourselves

1 Check in with yourself, **everyday.**

2 **Accept** how you feel and how you are.

3 **Meet** your needs, **don't** judge them.

4 Always try to **learn** more about yourself. Expand your horizons. Look for new opportunities. Keep your eyes open.

The goals you set should be TRUE TO YOURSELF. As you become your own best friend, you will learn more about your likes and dislikes. Use this knowledge to set goals for yourself and to choose your path. Don't choose a path that you **should** do, choose the path that fits.

This leads directly to the next guideline.

5. **Accept yourself as a permanent work in progress. Remember to use life as an opportunity to learn, not as something you win or lose.**

Hopefully, the meaning of these guidelines is clearer. Maybe you have actually been practicing some of these strategies, and things are starting to click. Maybe your motivation is now up to start trying some of this stuff. The point is, if you are being your own best friend and treating yourself as an honored guest, you are listening to yourself. If you are listening to yourself, you are learning more about yourself. If you are learning more about yourself, the goals that you set for yourself naturally follow. Take a few minutes (O.K. perhaps quite a few minutes) and think about the goals and standards you set for yourself and why you set them. Think about your expectations of yourself regarding your role as parent, spouse, friend, employee, etc. Ask yourself the following questions:

Three Key Questions:

Is this goal helping me to grow and learn (as opposed to interfering with my health and well-being)?

Does this goal suit me (i.e. is it consistent with my personal values and desires)?

Is this a goal I would be comfortable if my child adopted it?

If the goal passes, it's a keeper. If it fails the test, we will teach you how to tweak it so you can help your child.

Helping Your Child Become a Professional

How can you assist your child in rechanneling perfectionism into professionalism? We provide you with three steps.

1. Start with what you control: yourself.

As we have emphasized throughout this program, your example is a powerful one. It is really important that you take a step back and take an honest look at your current approach to mistakes and the strategies you use to set personal goals. Can you accept feedback without shame or guilt? Are you taking good care? Remember, don't use whether you achieve the goal as your metric. Instead, ask yourself "At what cost do I achieve this goal?" If a goal causes you to sacrifice health, happiness, and well-being, it is not an appropriate goal, even if you sometimes achieve it. Unless this happens, your child may be confused regarding appropriate limits.

Tip Box: Fears of Growing Up

Many individuals with eating disorders struggle with fears about becoming an adult. Part of this fear may stem from their difficulty in setting limits for themselves. Without this skill, the demands of adulthood can indeed seem overwhelming. As parents and adults, we symbolize what adulthood is like. Think about what your child may think about what adulthood means if we are always tired, burned out, stressed, etc. It's sad that modern society's pull is for everyone to be "crazy busy." However, we choose whether we follow along or stay true to what is best for us. It will greatly help your child to see what healthy limits look like.

---

2. Be consistent in your messages when your child makes a mistake.

Simply, if we panic when our child makes a mistake or harp for 10 years about what he should have done differently, we convey that mistakes are horrible. Don't forget the important steps we have learned about behavior management:

1   Praising the baby steps toward the goals spurs motivation to take further steps toward the goal. Always comparing to the outcome may create helplessness and hopelessness. Think: Mouse in the Maze.
2   There is a time to praise and a time to teach. Give advice when it is asked for.

3. Don't forget the wave.

So how can you help your child? Well one way is to help her think through her own goals through discussions and support. When you catch your child getting frustrated or when your child has just been riding the emotional wave, it may be because she is frustrated with herself for violating a rule. **AFTER THE INTENSITY OF THE WAVE HAS PASSED,** set up a time to talk about it.

Here's an example:
PARENT: Why did you get so frustrated at yourself before?
CHILD: I was sitting in the waiting room at the eating disorder program, and everyone there was skinnier than me.

PARENT: Comparing yourself to others really seems to upset you and interfere with your confidence. I didn't deal with that situation when I was your age, but I did struggle with comparing myself to my friends in terms of boyfriends. If you feel like talking about, I'd be happy to share some strategies.
CHILD: Mom, that's really dumb. What did you do?

Tip Box: Communicating with an Adolescent Revisited
Children, particularly adolescents (and spouses), will rarely acknowledge anything you do is helpful, at all. However, that does not mean you haven't planted an important seed that will grow when ready.

In addition, beware of jumping on the wave with him. If you do, you inadvertently communicate what your child is worried about deserves that degree of upset. Instead, wait patiently on the beach. Then talk.

4. Set Limits When Necessary

Don't forget, individuals with eating disorders present parents with a challenging dilemma: they often do too much of a good thing. We have no trouble imposing limits if our child asked us to take drugs, commit a crime, engage in risky sexual behavior; but studying? Practicing a musical instrument? Practicing athletics? Aren't these things they are asked to do? YES, in MODERATION. Many individuals with eating disorders have extreme difficulty switching on the "off" button and thus their goals break the guidelines; they interfere with health. Sometimes parents have to step in and set the limit when their child cannot set his own. With drugs the path is just clearer but the message is the same. Your children will certainly protest in the moment – that is their job – to push limits. However, that does not mean they do not feel safer because of the limit; they do.

5. Avoid the Perfectionism Traps

We've just given you a lot of information. We next present some situations along with some PERFECTIONISM TRAPS. These traps are SUBTLE things that parents do with the best of intentions that may accidentally convey the message that BEING PERFECT IS VERY IMPORTANT. Make it into a game. See who has fallen into the most traps in your family.

Situation #1: Your child comes to you and speaks about a problem she is having. Careful, don't fall into the...

Perfectionism Trap: "The Perfect Parent Trap." The job of parents is to help children learn, not to try to fix everything. **To escape the trap:** Listen, don't try to fix it unless your child wants advice. Often parents struggle with their own brand of perfectionism and this may include being a "perfect parent." Part of this belief may be that a perfect parent would fix all their children's problems. Well, in brief, this just isn't true. Children SO VALUE being listened to. Further, we often help them most when we help them to help themselves than when we try to save them.

INSTEAD, when you have a conversation with your child, make your focus the conversation itself. Your goal is simply to fully participate in the conversation by listening to what your child has to say and trying to figure out your child's position.

If you are confused whether your child wants advice or wants you to listen, just ask!! "Do you want my advice or do you just want me to listen?"

Escaping the trap.....

> Leslie and I had a fight at school today. She borrowed my books and didn't return them so I asked for them back and she got mad.

> Well, that stinks. I am sorry she made you feel badly when you were just asking for what is yours. I hate it when my friends do that to me.

Situation #2: Your child is in a sad mood. Careful. Don't fall into the ....
Perfectionism Trap: The limits of control trap.

To escape the trap: Take responsibility for what is yours. ONLY. Remember our Perfectionism Myth #5 in which we spoke about the things we have control over and the things we don't? The answer I am looking for is: "Of course I remember! I remember everything I read in this workbook." Well, a big trap many parents get stuck in is thinking that they are responsible for their child's emotions. They often feel that if their child is sad, mad, etc., it is their job to change their mood.

When your children were little, this **was** your job. Why? Well, emotions were the only form of communication your child had. As your children get older, your jobs change. Your job is to assist your child in decoding her own emotions, helping her think through the need communicated by these emotions, and modeling or suggesting ways to meet that need skillfully via your example and if asked for your advice. Taking responsibility for something that you can't control can be NERVEWRACKING. Thus, I often see parents get very frustrated or panicky when their child gets upset. This makes sense if you believe that it is your responsibility to cheer them up. I am giving you official permission to help them use their emotions to help them figure things out. PRESSURE IS OFF. NO FIXING FOR YOU.

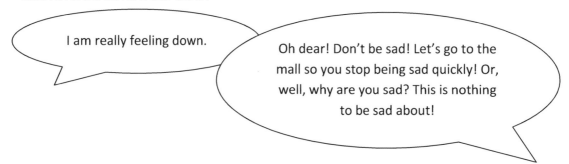

> I am really feeling down.

> Oh dear! Don't be sad! Let's go to the mall so you stop being sad quickly! Or, well, why are you sad? This is nothing to be sad about!

How? First, <u>acknowledge and describe their mood. Let them know it is OK and understandable to feel that way.</u> Your children have the right to feel however they choose to feel. They need to know this. Then, help them to understand what their mood is communicating to them, if they are in a mindset to talk about it.

Being sad, mad, anxious are normal, natural events. Rather than trying to change your child's mood, help your child learn to listen to her emotions so she can learn what her emotions are communicating. Certainly, you can offer helpful suggestions and role model how you handle your own emotions. What is not as helpful is if you feel so much pressure to keep your children happy that it makes you anxious when they are upset. When this happens, your child can get panicky about being upset and the emotional waves start rolling.   No worries. We spend the entire next chapter addressing emotions.

> Do you feel like talking about what happened earlier? Good. Let's try to figure out what your sadness is telling you that you need. I know when I'm sad, I often need support from someone…

It is very powerful when parents can remain calm and thoughtful in the face of negative emotions.

Situation #3: Your child brings home a grade that is less than optimal according to your rulebook. Careful. Don't fall into the…

Perfectionism Trap: "Yes, But" Trap.

To escape the trap: Applaud current accomplishments and stop there. We as parents accidentally fall into this trap whenever our child is sharing a goal or outcome and our response is something like "great job, BUT maybe next time…" This trap makes a lot of sense. As parents, we try to teach our children new things and guide them onward. However, there is a time and a place for this. They need to know that we are satisfied with what they do. PERIOD. Save teaching for another time. Otherwise, we give the message that nothing they ever do is good enough. A recipe for perfectionism.

Your child prepares a science project in which you notice many mistakes and your child has not asked for help – just approval.

> How do you like my science project?   Isn't it great?   I am really proud of it.

> It's wonderful. I really like this part here where you drew the frog.

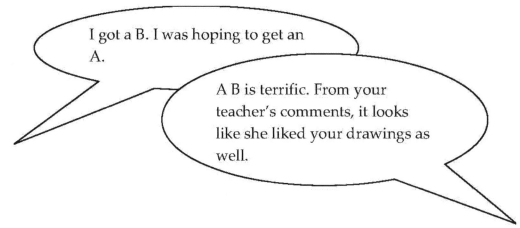

The next time your child works on a project, you can refer her to the teacher's comments so she can use these comments as a chance to learn. However, odds are, with your positive feedback, she is motivated to work harder because her baby steps felt so rewarding!

Situation: Your child complains about something you did that hurt her feelings. Careful. Don't fall into the …

Perfectionism Trap: "Sorry, but" Trap. This trap occurs whenever we have difficulty just accepting feedback or apologizing. Instead, we give excuses or defend our position. This inadvertently sends the message that we are never wrong and that errors are horrible.

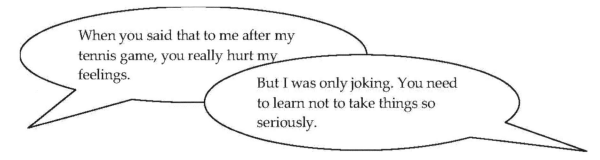

To escape the trap: Sometimes it is necessary to just take the feedback or just to say I'm sorry. Period.

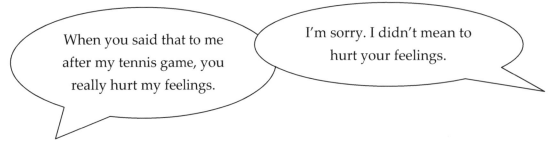

Situation: Your child is studying for a test and is getting very nervous. With the best of intentions, you tell your child, don't worry about the test. Just do your best. Whoops!! You have just fallen into the…

Perfectionism Trap: "Just do your best." What is the "do your best" trap? Well, as you have learned, your children are not good at setting limits for themselves. They are not good at listening to their own needs and responding to them. Instead, they push themselves way too hard. To tell them to "DO THEIR BEST" is not helpful because in their mind, their "best" is working around the clock, exercising until they drop.

To escape the trap: Communicate your lack of concern about their achievement through your actions and words. Assert again and again that their health is most important. Help them to set reasonable guidelines for study time, bed time, extracurricular activity time.

Situation: Your family is sitting around the dinner table talking about Johnny the Math Wiz, Susie the Soccer Star, Gina the Gymnast.

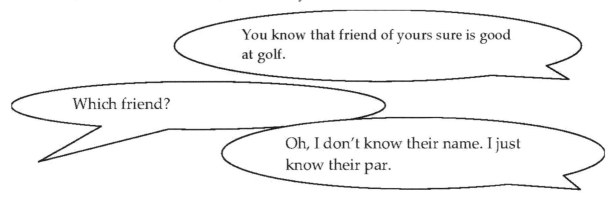

UH-OH! You have just fallen into the…

Perfectionism Trap: "You are what you do."

Oftentimes, individuals with eating disorders struggle with the notion of what makes a person special. They often think that others are special based on what THEY DO as opposed to WHO THEY ARE. They have a difficult time grasping that all people are special and unique because we are all an interesting combination of our likes, dislikes, annoying habits, special quirks, personality features and mannerisms. Instead, individuals with an eating disorder often define people based on tangible things. Thus, you often hear them express fears such as "If I am not the top of my class then I won't be special."

To escape the trap: It is important when you discuss your children and others that you mention both intrinsic qualities as well as extrinsic features. Then the importance of these features is clear.

Key Points.

1. If you struggle with perfectionism, you came by it honestly. It's certainly not your fault that you are here, but your children are depending on you to teach both yourself and them a more effective way.

2. Apply your process focus to how you set goals and handle setbacks.

3. Use your knowledge of yourself to inform the goals you choose.

4. Role model and teach these strategies to your children.

5. Be wary of subtle perfectionism traps.

6. Learn, learn, learn…and laugh.

Questions and Answers.

Q: I agree with a lot of what you said. It is my spouse that is the problem. What do I do about him/her?
A: That is tough. I hope that both of you are reading this book together. If not, all you can do is convey how important it is that he/she read it also because it would mean a great deal to your child. As you well know, we will often do for our child what we won't do for ourselves.

Q: I don't think this applies to my child. My child's problem is she doesn't live up to her potential and doesn't push herself hard enough. What should I do in this situation?
A: Careful. You may have a hidden perfectionist on your hands. Remember that part of perfectionism is procrastination. This looks like a topic of a good conversation as you both explore together why she has trouble approaching tasks. A fear of not doing well is often the root of much avoidance.

Wisdom of the Week: My Gift to Myself

I think you could use a good laugh, don't you? I think a girl's night or guy's night out may be just the ticket.

Date:

Remember our key guidelines

It's a process! Try, tweak, grow and learn.

Self-parenting: a necessary prerequisite for other parenting.

Learn how to SURF The WAVE!

Remain genuine.

Unhealthy or unhelpful behavior I will discuss WITH my child this week and our plan to address it.

Eats too little	Eats too little variety	Exercises too much
Throws up after meals	Doesn't get enough sleep	Doesn't set limits
Abuses laxatives	Engages in self-harm	Other

Possible Suggestions of How to Address:	My Plan:
☐ Ignore it ☐ Have a discussion about needed change in behavior *(discuss a future, necessary, logical consequence given the severity of the behavior)* ☐ Implement a logical consequence (reminding your child of the importance of health before anything) ☐ Appeal to your child's inner wisdom (have a discussion with your child about what you have observed, why you are concerned, the change in behavior expected) ☐ Reverse Time-Out (you leave) ☐ Group Time-Out (everyone leaves for 10 minutes) ☐ Regrouping (family meeting to get out of power struggle) ☐ Humor	Would a discussion be a good idea?

Heathy Coping Strategy I will address with my child this week and my plan to address it.

Express negative emotions effectively	Ask for more help	Set more limits (cut down study time, set a regular bedtime, cut out an activity)
Express an opinion- even if someone may disagree	Be more considerate of others	Place more realistic demands on oneself (consider the cost, not whether the demands are achieved)
Get a better balance of work and leisure	View a situation with curiosity rather than with criticism	Manage disappointing results
Share a vulnerability with someone	Embrace and learn from mistakes rather than running from them	Resolve a conflict
Tune in and respond more to what your feelings are telling you	Take more pride in oneself (being a more respectful self-parent)	Strut
Be Silly or just take yourself less seriously	Smile at your reflection	Initiate plans
Try something new	Get Messy	Break a ritual
Get more sleep	Other	Other

Possible Suggestions:	My Plan:
☐ Positive attention when takes a step toward behavior ☐ One-on-one time outside of eating disorder stuff ☐ Earning a logical privilege given increased health ☐ Praise and STOP – no BUTS ☐ Role Model Behavior Yourself ☐ Open the door for a discussion ☐ Set a limit ☐ Offer to teach ☐ Other	

Heathy Coping Strategy I will Role Model this week.

Possible Suggestions:	My Plan:
☐ Delegate something. ☐ Say 'no' to some things. ☐ Be honest with my feelings. ☐ Express my feelings when not on the wave. ☐ Ask for help. ☐ Set healthy limits between my needs and those of others. ☐ Listen with full attention. ☐ Praise and STOP. ☐ Say "I'm sorry" with no excuses. ☐ Allow family members to make mistakes without jumping in. ☐ Be consistent. ☐ Address negative self-talk. ☐ Be reliable.	

Self-care Strategy I will implement this week

Possible Suggestions:	My Plan:
☐ Make regular mealtimes a priority. ☐ Set a regular bedtime. ☐ Learn a new hobby. ☐ Spend some time with my friends. ☐ Spend time ALONE with my spouse. ☐ Set a regular time I stop work each day. ☐ Take weekends off. ☐ Buy something for myself. ☐ Exercise in a MODERATE manner. ☐ Take pride in my physical appearance.	No lame excuses!!

TIP OF THE WEEK: No buts. Stick to process.

CHAPTER FOURTEEN: Fine-tuning the Emotional Wave

Where You Are

✓ Time for more advanced work. We are about to take our skill with the emotional wave one step further. We need to get more comfortable with figuring out what upset us in the first place and taking steps to address these factors.

Key Messages

It's a process: try, tweak, learn, grow.

"Self-parenting" is a necessary step for "other parenting."

Stay off the WAVE.

Remain genuine.

Topic: The Advanced Emotional Wave

In this chapter, we take skills you already have (your emotional wave skills) and help you bring them to an advanced level. Before we "dive" in (sorry, couldn't resist) to learning new things, we would like to spend several moments discussing why emotions are so important. Many individuals with eating disorders don't think that emotions are important at all and go to unhealthy lengths to ignore the very existence of their feelings. You may have a certain fear of emotions yourself. Hopefully we can help you to understand why it is important to feel comfortable with your feelings and help you to not be so intimidated.

To really understand feelings, we need to go back to the beginning and think about the relationship between a parent and a child. Pull out a baby picture, and we'll get started.

In the beginning.

When a child is an infant, their emotional displays are their only form of communication because they can't talk. Think about the interaction between a parent and infant. The baby cries. Parents respond to the crying with different strategies until the infant stops crying. Several things happen as a result of this back and forth parent-child interaction.

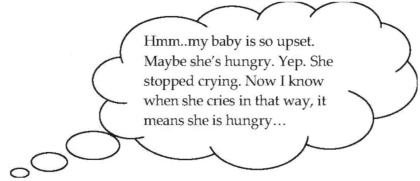

Hmm..my baby is so upset. Maybe she's hungry. Yep. She stopped crying. Now I know when she cries in that way, it means she is hungry…

1. The parent **learns something** about his baby.
For example, when the baby cries, and the parent does something that ends the crying, the parent has just acquired some new knowledge about what the child likes and does not like.

2. The child's emotions help to **guide our actions.**
Our child's emotions help to guide the actions we take. For example, if our child is happy we will pursue a different course of action than if she is upset or angry. Emotions help tell us what actions we need to take.

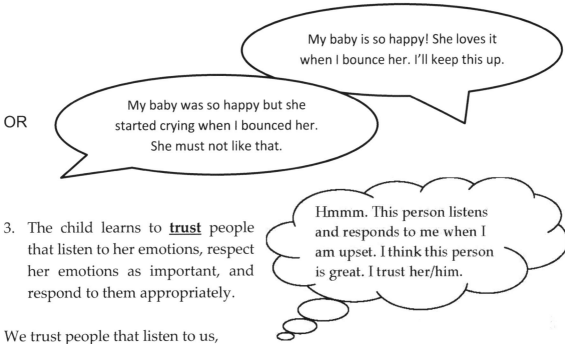

My baby is so happy! She loves it when I bounce her. I'll keep this up.

OR

My baby was so happy but she started crying when I bounced her. She must not like that.

3. The child learns to **trust** people that listen to her emotions, respect her emotions as important, and respond to them appropriately.

Hmmm. This person listens and responds to me when I am upset. I think this person is great. I trust her/him.

We trust people that listen to us, validate us, and take steps to help us. This is what happens when a parent responds to her baby's emotional expressions. Keep this in mind as we think about what happens as your children get older.

As time goes on..... The child's emotional displays and the parent's response helps the parent get to know her child. As young infants don't have the ability to reason (or talk), emotions are their only form of communication and the messages they are sending are not complicated. I'm hungry. I'm tired. Pay attention to me. I need to cuddle.

With growth and maturity two things happen. First, life gets more complicated. Thus, one emotion can mean **many, many different things**. Thus, in order for us to understand our child's needs she needs to learn other forms of communication. Second, your children need to take on the task of regulating their own emotions. Our job is to teach them how and to help and support them in this task. Your child may have been OK at managing her emotions and the disorder threw her off balance or she may have never been very good. In either case, we'll help to get her back on track. Don't worry about how. We'll show you.

Why is it important for our children to learn to manage their own emotions? Think about the important things we just learned about emotions.

> They give us information.
> They guide our actions.
> When we listen and respond to them we build trust.

When your child learns to listen to and respond to her emotions, she gets these important benefits.

She starts to learn about herself.
She begins to trust herself.
Her emotions help guide her actions.

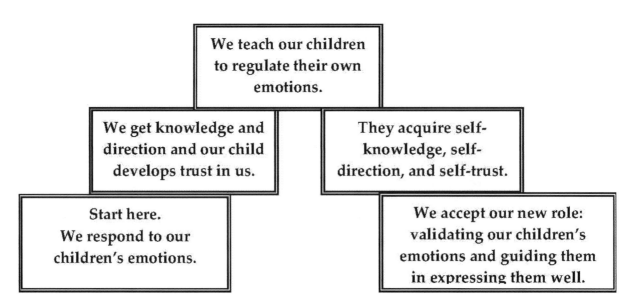

We teach our children to regulate their own emotions.

We get knowledge and direction and our child develops trust in us.

They acquire self-knowledge, self-direction, and self-trust.

Start here.
We respond to our children's emotions.

We accept our new role: validating our children's emotions and guiding them in expressing them well.

HOW do we teach our children to regulate their emotions? Well, we can't very well teach things that we are not comfortable with ourselves. First, we have to make sure we are comfortable with managing OUR emotions. Then we can help our children. We need to go through these steps.

- We learn more about and get comfortable managing our own emotions.
- We get comfortable acknowledging the emotions of our children (without feeling that we have to do something about them).
- We guide our children in the use of emotion regulation strategies.
- We accept our limits.

Step One: We learn more about and get comfortable managing our own emotions

Just when you think you finally had it mastered, we are going to get a little fancier. We have to go back to our emotional wave and figure out what to do once you get yourself down from the wave. By now, you are very familiar with the emotional wave. Maybe you have become better at recognizing the stage of the wave you are on. Maybe you are better at getting yourself down from the wave before you react. Maybe you are more comfortable when others are riding the wave. Maybe you have achieved all these things. Now, it's time to take things a step further. We have talked about the need to go back to the beginning of the wave and figure out what bothered you in the first place. Now we are going to take that step more seriously. It's time to learn what to do once you have gotten yourself down from the top of the wave.

Remember our simple formula?

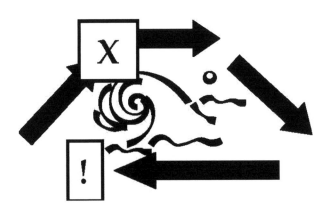

Step 3. You have come down from the wave. However, if you don't go back and figure out what your emotion was telling you, you won't get the benefits (no direction, no self-knowledge, no self-trust) AND the need won't be

All the answers
are here!

Going back to the beach. Why you can't avoid it.

Our emotions give us a message. A message that will not be ignored (even if we try really hard to ignore it). Emotions are a signal that something is going on. In order for us to benefit from this message and develop a sense of self-trust, we have to listen to this message and respond to it. Then the message is delivered and the emotion will end, or decrease. That's emotion regulation in a nutshell! Of course, it's more difficult in practice, but understanding this basic concept is important. Emotion regulation involves calmness, patience, and thoughtfulness, not a top of the wave task to be sure! So, our first job is to get off the wave. Then, we can investigate what this emotion is trying to tell us.

Confused? Think about this example. You have plans with a friend. She cancels plans at the last minute which is very frustrating because you had rearranged your whole afternoon to be with her. She has also done this before. Several times. You do a great job of coming off the wave and your anger is under control, BUT...if you don't go back and tell her about what she does that upsets you, then your anger will not end. It is bubbling below the surface and the next time you interact with her, it will take even less to go to the top of the wave........

The Ideal World Scenario

> Jeanie, we need to talk. I have to say I was very disappointed when you cancelled plans the other day. I was really looking forward to seeing you. The next time that happens, will you please give me more notice? This way, I won't get my hopes up and will have time to fill my schedule with other plans.

> I am really sorry about that. The problem is my organization. I need to get more organized so other things don't interfere with my plans. I'll work on that. I miss seeing you too.

emotions will be to manage and the better you will get to know yourself.

☀ Perfectionist's Corner ☀

Perfectionist: But if I go back to what upset me in the first place, I'll get upset all over again.

Voice of Reason: Yes, I can understand that it is hard to go back and talk about what was bothering you. You are right. It may make you and the other person involved (if there is one), get upset all over again. However, there are two things to think about. First, we need practice in managing negative emotions. Thus, the more you talk about them and work through them, the more comfortable you'll get with feelings. As you practice, going back and figuring out what upset will get less and less scary.

The second thing to think about is our feelings about feelings. Feeling sad, angry, anxious, etc. is an important part of life. Once you start listening and getting more comfortable with your feelings, you'll realize that feelings are what they are. No more. No less. They give information. They help us learn. They make life joyous. They hurt a whole lot sometimes. The more comfortable you get with feelings, the easier your emotions will be to manage and the better you will get to know yourself.

Figuring out when

So how do you figure out what put you on the wave in the first place? Well, you have to play detective. Even if you think you know what upset you, it is usually a good idea to do a little thinking. We aren't always upset or angry for the obvious reasons. Sometimes we need to do a little snooping. A good place to start is the beginning of the day. I usually instruct the people I work with to do a "chain analysis" to figure out at what point in the day their mood shifted; either from good to bad or from bad to worse.

A chain analysis is a play-by-play analysis of your day. Your goal is to figure out what was upsetting you by isolating the period of the day when your mood shifted. We will walk you through a sample chain analysis below.

It usually goes something like this:

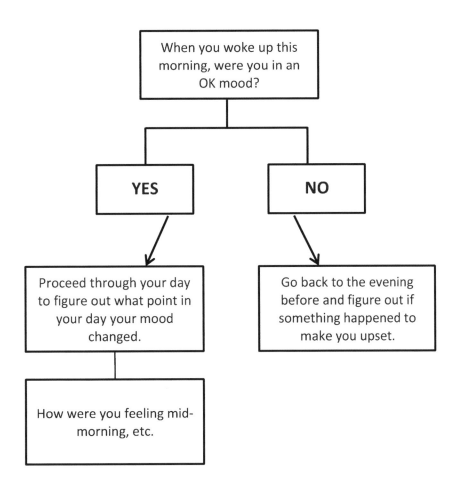

…and so on. Your goal is to pinpoint the time of the day that your mood changed from good to bad, from bad to worse, etc.

Figuring out what

After you have figured out the point in the day when you mood shifted, your next step is to figure out WHAT upset you. Basically, there are three things that could have happened.

- You have a problem with something about yourself.
- You have a problem with someone else.
- You have a problem with a situation.

That really about covers all the topics!

There are different strategies to deal with each of these situations. Let's walk you through each scenario.

When the WHAT is YOU.

You figure out the point in the day where your mood changed and what happened during that time.

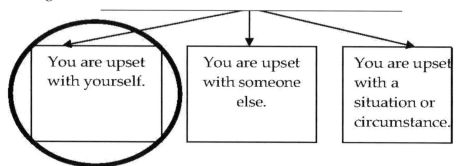

You may be angry at something you did or didn't do or you may be dissatisfied with some aspect of yourself. Because of this, you may have entered into the bottomless cavern of negative self-criticism and now you feel horrible.

What should you do?

RUN, do not walk, quickly back to your process approach towards yourself.

From here, we are in a more logical place where we can consider our options.

Scenario 1: You are upset with something you DID or DID NOT do.

OPTION 1.   Reframe whatever happened as an opportunity for learning.

- Think about what you learned from the experience.
- Plan what you would do differently next time.
- Pat yourself on the back for making the best decision you knew how to at the time (no sense in blaming yourself for what you have learned since that time; that's not fair).
- Accept what you did, learn from it, move on.

OPTION 2. Give yourself a break.

Remember our distinction between process-generated rules and outcome-focused rules? Process-focused rules meet three criteria: a) They take our own needs and strengths into account; b) They don't sacrifice our health or well-being; c) They are rules that we would be comfortable if our children followed.

Given this, make sure you are not angry or upset with yourself for failing to follow an outcome-focused rule. If you are, stop beating yourself up! JUST CHANGE THE RULE!

Scenario 2: You are upset with something about yourself AS A PERSON.

OPTION 1. Remember your process approach. You are always an excellent "work in progress". Accept what you cannot change. Change what you can. You will have yourself until you die. Thus, it would certainly make life more worth living if you enjoyed your own company. Hopefully, each day you will work on strengthening your relationship with yourself, getting to know yourself, and treating yourself as an honored guest. Part of this process is accepting yourself as you are in the current moment while seeking to grow and learn more about yourself. Am I contradicting myself? No, the message is "I am super as I am, and I can always learn more."

Put on your reporter's hat. Describe the situation you are upset about by sticking to the facts (in other words, don't let your feelings and opinions cloud how you view the situation). After you have done this, is there something you can work on so you handle the situation better the next time? Make a plan of how to address it. Now you're in familiar territory. Try out the plan. See how it goes. Tweak it. Try again.

> Hello self. Well, I guess you're all I've got so I may as well work with you. I do think you're kind of cute. I know we can work on that annoying habit you have of leaving a trail of papers behind you...

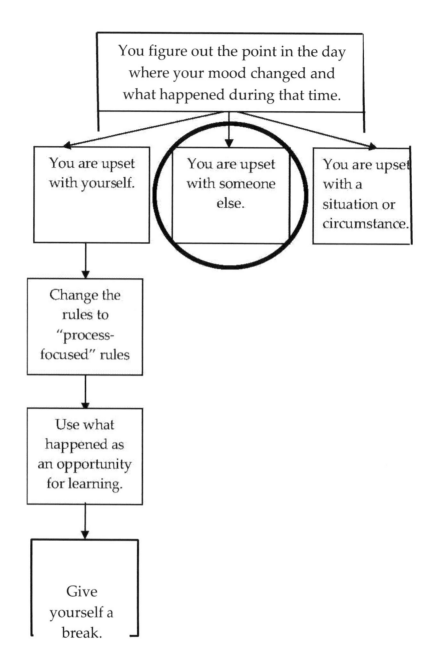

When the WHAT is SOMEONE ELSE.

Did the situation involve someone else? If so, there are two steps we'll have to take. First, we will need to think through the interaction and figure out what the other person did that bothered us. Next, we will have to talk to them about it.

However, there are effective ways to talk to someone and ways that don't work as well. To do this, we'll brush up on our communication skills. Communication skills deserve their own Chapter so we talk about talking in Chapter 15.

When the WHAT is a SITUATION.

Here is where our acceptance and change skills come into play. We have to examine the situation and separate the elements of the situation we can do something about from those elements of the situation that are beyond our control. We need to channel our energy into those aspects of the situation

that we can change and work on accepting those aspects of the situation that are beyond our reach. Life presents us with unexpected challenges. Some of these challenges are indescribably awful.

However, our process approach has taught us that we need to work with the journey we are on, not the one we wish we were traveling! I found a very thought-provoking quote by a psychologist named Jon Kabat-Zinn in his wonderful book *Full Catastrophe Living.* Dr. Zinn uses mindfulness approaches (similar in some ways to our process approach) to help patients learn to accept and manage their chronic pain.

> You are upset with a situation or circumstance.

> You are upset with a situation or circumstance.

> Approach the person with impeccable communication skills.

> Use your emotions to guide the change that is needed.

The quote is: ***"Pain is inevitable. Suffering is optional."*** In other words, rather than wishing a situation were different, and thereby increasing our suffering, we can work on accepting the pain that is a part of life and become increasingly skilled at working through pain. Doing so brings growth and meaning from pain, not suffering.

Wishing a situation is different than the way it is, is human, but may not be helpful. It's not helpful if this "wishing" gets in the way of our ability to deal with the situation at hand. BOTTOM LINE: We may not always like the situations we find ourselves in. In fact, they may be downright awful. However, wishing things were different only increases suffering. Instead, accepting and working with your current journey will not only decrease suffering, it will also facilitate your growth as a person.

How to begin? Well, first we need to act like an investigative reporter. Huh???? Stay with me for a moment. The job of an investigative reporter is to observe and describe. Just the facts, ma'am. Why? Well because reporters are supposed to present stories in an unbiased fashion. Opinions bias what we see.

EXAMPLE: I hate beef stew (this is a true story).

If I go into a meal with this opinion in the forefront of my mind, I am not going to give beef stew a fair shot. I will focus on how dry the meat is, how unpleasantly squishy the potatoes are, rather than the delicious savory smell of the beef broth.

POINT: If we act like an investigative reporter, we can get a better handle of the situation we have to deal with because we are describing it without bias. We will more likely see what there is to see.

Once we have a factual description of the situation, we have to determine what aspects of the situation we have the power to change and which aspects we don't.

When aspects of the situation are beyond our control

For the aspects of the situation we can change, we brainstorm and create a plan to change it. We try it. We see how it goes. We learn. We tweak it. We try again. For a situation that we need to accept, we need our wave skills to help keep our mind clear and effective. We can use any of the skills from our toolbox to manage the distress of dealing with a situation we wish could be different.

Tip Box

A powerful strategy to cope with a situation you do not have control over is to find meaning. Very cruel, unfair things happen in this world. Often our only option in situations such as that is to use that moment as a springboard for efforts to make the world a better place to live. For example, one of the mothers I worked with decided to go spend a few hours a week at a soup kitchen. She had so lost the joy of eating that she wanted to be in a situation in which she was with others who truly valued the wonder of having something to eat. It worked.

Let's spend some time looking at a few emotions so you can get a better idea of what we mean.

The Messages of Emotions

To be an advanced surfer, it is important to understand emotions. If you do, you may lose any fear you have either of your own or the emotions of others as understanding is often an important first step in approaching discomfort. To truly understand emotions, remember this key point: **emotions are messengers**. Each type of emotion sends us a message of a need that we have. Different emotions send different messages and thus communicate different needs. Understanding the message of your emotions is the key to emotion regulation. For this to really make sense, consider some examples.

Emotion: Sadness

Potential message: "I need comfort and support."

Ways to respond to the message: Well, you need to get comfort and support. First, you have to give yourself permission (no guilt please) to engage in "recuperative withdrawal" (I love that term. I picked it up from Dr. Leslie Greenberg an expert in emotion regulation). Recuperative withdrawal is when you give yourself permission to withdraw from activities and responsibilities because you just don't have the energy for them. Instead, you need to step back and take care of yourself. Or you may need to seek support from someone else.

 Perfectionist's Corner ✿

Perfectionist: But if I allow myself to withdraw from activities, I'll get behind. Or what if relaxing feels so good I never want to go back and do the things I used to do? What if I can never muster my energy again?

Voice of Reason: Whoa there! Not so fast. First of all, when we push ourselves to the limit, we get tired. When we are tired, we are less efficient. Things take longer. Thus stopping to rest and relax makes us MORE efficient. If we stop and rest, not only do we not get behind, we get caught up.

Secondly, this may be a good time for you to evaluate your priorities. If you are dreading going back to the way things were, then it is time to make some changes. Responsibilities should be balanced by relaxation. If not, what's the point? When needs for rest or relaxation are not responded to, sadness creeps in. If this goes on, perhaps sadness becomes deep sadness like depression. For some of the people I work with, when they are depressed is the only time they give themselves permission to slow down. Listen to sadness. Take care of yourself. You're worth it. Resting bring energy and renewed efforts -not laziness.

Emotion: Anger

Potential message: "Someone or something has violated my rights."

Ways to respond to the message: With anger, there is usually a need to communicate with someone else regarding something they did or did not do that hurt our feelings. We need to tell them what they did and ask for changes.

Tip Box

MOST people are not great at receiving feedback in the MOMENT. It takes practice. People may get very defensive or argue. HOWEVER, don't despair. Even if it doesn't seem like they got anything out of what you said, you may have planted a small seed that may blossom and grow into an effective person. What you can work on is the manner in which you give feedback to minimize the likelihood that this will happen (This goes back to the communication skills we will discuss in the next chapter).

✸ Perfectionist's Corner ✸

Perfectionist: But if I tell someone I am angry with them, I may hurt their feelings and it may damage the relationship.

Voice of Reason: If you tell someone about something he or she did that made you angry, it may hurt her feelings (especially if she is not an expert on receiving feedback like you are). However, she'll get over it. The cost of not doing it is just too great; it may end the relationship. As unexpressed anger builds, relationships start to sour and are not genuine anyway! The more comfortable you get giving and receiving feedback, the stronger the relationship will grow. It's an amazingly comfortable and freeing feeling when you can be honest with others about your feelings and know that the relationship is strong enough to handle it.

Emotion: Anxiety

Potential message: "There is POTENTIAL danger."

Ways to respond to the message: The word POTENTIAL here is very important. With anxiety, our first job is to determine whether our worry thoughts are <u>helpful</u> or <u>unhelpful.</u> Sometimes our anxiety is misguided. In other words, we get anxious when the likelihood of threat is very small. Before we can decide what needs to be done, we first have to distinguish helpful worries from unhelpful worries. What's the difference? Of course, we have a diagram.

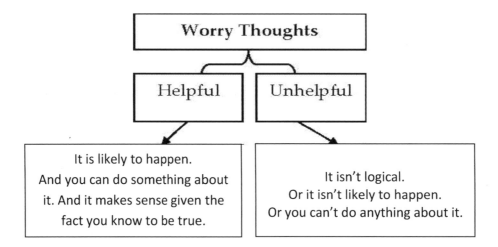

Let's start with the unhelpful worries.

To understand how to deal with unhelpful worries, we have to speak for a few moments about thoughts. The American Heritage dictionary defines a thought as a "mental conception, whether an opinion, judgment, idea, etc. Thoughts are essentially words (or images) that pass through our minds. They can reflect our beliefs, our history, a random thing that popped into our head because it was distantly associated with another thing, a wish, gibberish, and on and on.

What is important to know is that you CANNOT CONTROL what your thoughts say. They are random. For example, if you are really worried about something, you can't just say "Stop thinking about such and so." That will never work. It would just make you think about it more! However, what you CAN do is change your RELATIONSHIP to your thoughts. You control how you RESPOND and MANAGE the thoughts you do have. You can take away their power so thoughts do not bother you as much. How?

1. Exercise your mind.

You can practice focusing your attention on specific things for set periods of time. Think of this as "brain calisthenics." The more you exercise your mind, the better you can get at shifting your attention from annoying thoughts. The thoughts will still come, but they won't be as distracting.

2. Question the power of thoughts.

If you think thoughts are powerful, that the mere occurrence of a thought is a premonition of what is sure to be, that a thought is an order or a mandate of what you must do, then of course <u>worry thoughts</u> would scare you! In fact, given what we have learned about thoughts, we know that none of these things are true. If that were true, I would think "I am rich, I am rich, I live on an island, and I live on an island. I am married to a famous movie star." Instead, we know that thoughts are just thoughts. Thoughts are random.

So how does this relate to worry thoughts? Well, you can't stop worry thoughts from going through your mind. However, just because a worry thought passes through your mind doesn't make it true, and if you view a worry thought as just random words that pass through your mind, the occurrence of the worry thought won't bother you as much.

Tip Box

I find it helpful to do just that: I picture the words of my thoughts and watch the words pass by in my mind. I watch them enter my left ear. I greet it. "Hello worry thought." I watch it pass over my forehead. I wave it goodbye. I watch it leave out of my right ear. I focus on what I am doing. I see it come again in my left ear. Greet it again….and so on. Another way to do this is to write your thoughts down. Thoughts change A LOT when they are down on paper than when they are running through your head.

This is actually a powerful strategy because it allows me to step back from my thoughts, observe them, decide whether they are helpful or unhelpful and go on from there.

How about helpful worries?

Well, by definition, you can DO SOMETHING about helpful worries. However, before you jump in, you first have to figure out what the problem is. A big problem with worry thoughts is that they are very general and don't really help to guide what we need to do. Familiar examples are:

> "I have so much to do."
> "I am so stressed out."
> "I'll never get everything done."
> "I can't handle this."

You know what I'm talking about... Thoughts like these do not give you any direction. They don't give you a good starting place. They don't tell you what problem needs to be solved. What you have to do first is <u>put words on the problem. Make it specific. The problem then becomes a tangible thing that you can get your mind around and begin to do something about.</u>

Here's an example.

> "I have so much to do."

O.K.

> What EXACTLY do I have to do?
> When does it need to be finished?
> What are some baby steps that I can break this problem into?

When you go through this process, you take this large global mass of worry and turn it into something you can take charge of. I can't tell you how much this process helps.

Tip Box
Plans that address things we can control help.
Plans that address things that we cannot control drive ourselves
and everyone else crazy!

Well, it could rain three months from now. Better start putting out the rain gear…

Enough said.

Emotion: Guilt
Potential message: "It is possible that I violated the rights of myself or others."
Ways to respond to the message: There are two situations that may be occurring when an individual experiences guilt.

1) We did something that hurt someone else (though we may not have meant to) and we need to do some repair work OR

2) We are too hard on ourselves. Our guilt is misplaced because our personal rules are the problem, not what we did or didn't do.

Here are some examples.

Situation 1

You messed up your schedule and missed an appointment with someone (yes, this is a personal example).

> La te dah.....Hmmm, I have this sinking feeling that I am supposed to be somewhere right now......

Solution: Yep. You goofed. Repair. Apologize. Take steps to change and MOVE ON. One apology is all that is needed. Just make sure the apology is sincere by making changes to avoid the reoccurrence of this situation.

Situation 2

A friend asks you to babysit her child. You have a million things you need to do and you just babysat for her last weekend. You say No, but you feel guilty about it. **Solution:** Change the rules. You have the right to say no. You have the right to put your needs first sometimes. It's about balance. If you always put the needs of others first, you sacrifice yourself. If you always put your own needs first, you sacrifice the quality of the relationship. Balance. Guess what? If you don't put your own needs first, you'll burn out and won't be able to help ANYONE.

Sigh, we've got a ways to go.....

Emotion: Shame

Potential message: There is a story that needs to be told and understood and there is a new ending to this story that needs to be written.

Ways to respond to the message. To understand the message of shame, first we need to understand shame. Shame is a powerful, extremely complex emotion. Whereas we feel guilt about something we **do,** shame is much deeper than that. Often when an individual feels shame, he or she has this deep sense there is something wrong with him or herself, as a person.

When I say shame has a story to tell, I mean that shame is a very complex emotion that develops as a result of someone's unique history. Understanding shame takes work and willingness. Thus, the first part of listening to the message of shame is tracing the trail of this story to understand the journey of this feeling for you.

There are some important things to understand before you pursue this story.

Often the seeds of shame are sown in childhood. When something happens to us as a child, we understand it as a child. Children cannot think abstractly; they think concretely and classify things simply. Things are black/white, right/wrong, good/bad, etc. Children are vulnerable and thus it is very important for children to feel safe. Often the explanations of situations they come up with make them feel safe, even at the expense of their own self-worth. Safety is that important. Consider this example. Suppose a parent was abusing a child. A child might think "I am very bad and deserve to be punished in this way." While not true, and while as adults we can recognize that it is the behavior of the adult that is blameworthy, this interpretation makes the child feel safer. It is safer for the child to be "bad" than for the parent to be "bad." Over time, this belief has just been around for so long that it just "feels true." And shame develops. Thus, to understand this feeling, this person would have to trace through that story and understand how the feeling developed and would rewrite the ending now that she has the interpretative capabilities of an adult. "She was not bad. Her parent was a very troubled individual."

Often the seed of shame are subtle. Subtle comments over time can also generate feelings of shame. As we have mentioned many times in this program, the essence of knowing and trusting oneself is reading the signals of one's body (hunger, emotion, fatigue) and responding to these signals. Shame can result if we are given the message that we are interpreting our signals incorrectly or if we are told the signals of our body are "wrong."

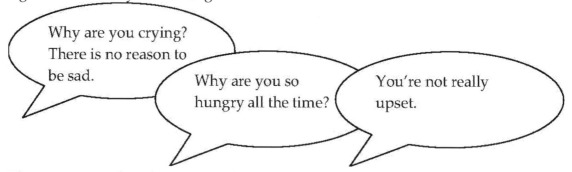

These are examples of comments that may inadvertently contribute to the development of shame over time in vulnerable individuals. It is terribly upsetting and confusing if our body is giving us certain signals and we are told those signals are wrong. If we need those signals to learn about ourselves, when someone tells us those signals are wrong, we just feel stuck and hopeless. Instead, we all need to accept and understand that only the person himself knows what he is feeling.

Shame can feel "truly deserved" not because it is deserved, but because we have thought this way for so long it just "seems" true.

As we mentioned, beliefs that we develop as children to make us feel safe stick around a long time. Thus, we may not question them as adults as it just "feels" true. Be aware of this and never be afraid to look with an open mind at one's history. We need to look at that history without judgment but rather with the knowledge that we all do the best we can at any given point in time given what we know and can do at that time. The ending we need to write as we cope with shame has to do with forgiveness and acceptance; acceptance that sometimes life can seem terribly unfair. And forgiveness, recognizing we all have an ugly and cruel side. As humans, we have some survival instincts that make us do and say hateful things. However, as humans we have the unique ability to transcend these instincts and use times of ugliness as times of growth. The hard part is that ugliness can come from within and it can come from without. We need to write an ending that helps us to gain understanding and forgiveness of ourselves and life's circumstances. Shame is such a deep-seeded emotion that you should not manage this one alone. Now is the time to turn to social support. People who truly know you can help you tell a different kind of story than the one you have weaved from your past.

Summary for Your Emotion Regulation
WHEW!!!!!! That's a lot of new stuff to learn. Let's review to make sure it makes sense. Right now we are working on **your** emotion regulation strategies so we can be in a better position to help our child manage his or her emotions.

STEPS

1. Get down from on top of the wave.

2. Go back and figure out what bothered you in the first place.

3. Take steps to improve the situation.

   -really that is all we are saying.

Why is this important?? Well, the benefits are **self-trust, self-knowledge, and guidance; and ultimately, self-confidence.**

Now for the kids

We have already introduced you to the eating disorder wave. Thus, hopefully you understand that although an "eating disorder event" may have **ultimately** triggered the wave for your child, other **key** issues sent him up the wave in the first place. These **real issues** made him more sensitive to later eating disorder issues. If you need a refresher, you may want to go back and reread this part in Chapter 3. Thus, when your child gets down from the wave, your child's job (with your help) is to figure out the **key issues** that sent him up the wave, not the eating disorder events. This takes practice. At first, your child may not accept this connection and may think it is all about a weight issue. You just have to trust us on this. The more your child goes through the steps we have outlined to figure out the "real" issue, the better he will get at it!

How can you help?

Tip Box

When the eating disorder is loud, help your child get off the wave.

Get through the current eating disorder situation (eat the meal, buy the outfit, pass by the mirror....the list, as you know, is endless).

Later, begin helping them to play detective to figure out the "true" problem.

Strategies to help your child learn to manage emotions

Strategy #1: **Introduce the connection between the volume of their eating disorder voice and distressful life events.**

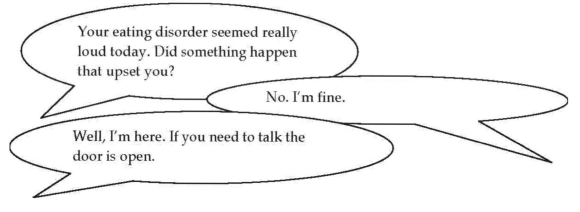

> Your eating disorder seemed really loud today. Did something happen that upset you?

> No. I'm fine.

> Well, I'm here. If you need to talk the door is open.

Even though this step may seem like it was useless, you've actually planted a very important seed. You have made an association between the volume of their eating disorder and a situation in their life.

Strategy #2: **Help them play detective to figure out what was really bothering them.**
There are two situations when your child's eating disorder is loud. Situation 1 is that they know what is wrong and don't feel like talking about it just then. Situation 2 is they don't really know what is wrong. For situation 1, the important thing is make sure you let your child know you are available, but don't PUSH IT. OFFER TO LISTEN and LET IT GO. She'll come to you when she's ready.

For situation 2, this is a useful strategy.

In an ideal world…

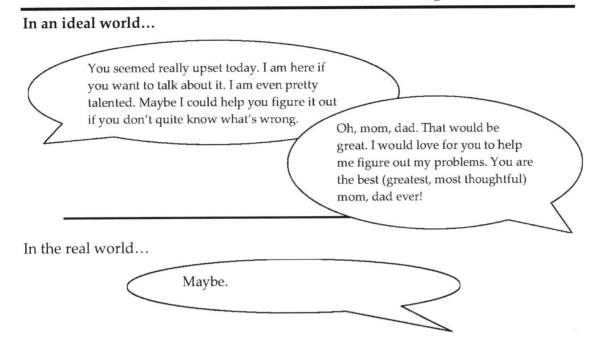

> You seemed really upset today. I am here if you want to talk about it. I am even pretty talented. Maybe I could help you figure it out if you don't quite know what's wrong.

> Oh, mom, dad. That would be great. I would love for you to help me figure out my problems. You are the best (greatest, most thoughtful) mom, dad ever!

In the real world…

> Maybe.

"Maybe" is actually adolescent speak for thanks.

So where do you begin when you've been given the go-ahead? You help your child play detective. Your mission is to help her walk through her day to figure out when her mood changed from good to bad or from bad to worse. Sound familiar? Yep. You're right. Now you're in familiar territory. These are the same steps you learned to manage your own emotions.

Tip Box

Figure out the problem.

Make a plan to address it.

Try it. See how it goes. Learn from it.

CONGRATULATIONS. YOU HAVE NOW MASTERED THE WAVE.

Key Points

1. The first and perhaps most important way for you to help your children get comfortable with their own emotions is to be comfortable with our own emotions.
2. Thus, our first goal is to master the emotional wave by going back to what upset us in the first place and figuring out what needs to be done.
3. The issue could be a problem with us, someone else, or a situation.
4. If with us, we need to figure out whether our behavior needs to be changed or our standards need to be changed.
5. If with someone else, we have to use good communication skills and knowledge about our emotions to guide our actions.
6. If a situation, we have to separate what we have control over versus what we do not. We need to practice change strategies with the former and acceptance strategies with the latter.
7. For our children, we have to understand the connection between their eating disorder and their emotions.
8. We need to help guild them in the use of strategies to get down from the wave and if the time is right, help them to figure out what is bothering them.

Questions and Answers

Q: What if I keep trying and my child is still not willing to talk to me about her problems? I can tell she is upset.

A: Patience is tough. Your best strategy is to keep opening the door for a conversation and let her walk through. You can't force someone to talk when they are not ready, and if you try, I promise the conversation won't go well. However, **sometimes** people are more comfortable communicating via one channel of communication over another. For example, some people prefer communicating over email versus talking in person. You might try sending your child an email and see how it goes. It may be a useful place to start.

Q: What if I can't figure out what is bothering my child?

A: If I didn't know better, I would say you were having an outcome focused moment. Stop that. The process of trying to figure what is going on is what is important. We never know if we are "right"; instead, we do some thinking. Come up with some likely possibilities and make some plans. Then we take it from there.

Gift to Myself

I do believe it is time to get away. For a day, for a weekend. Something.

You've been working very, very hard.

Date:

Remember our key guidelines
It's a process! Try, tweak, grow and learn.
Self-parenting: a necessary prerequisite for other parenting.
Learn how to SURF The WAVE!
Remain genuine.

Unhealthy or unhelpful behavior I will discuss WITH my child this week and our plan to address it.

Eats too little	Eats too little variety	Exercises too much
Throws up after meals	Doesn't get enough sleep	Doesn't set limits
Abuses laxatives	Engages in self-harm	Other

Possible Suggestions of How to Address:

☐ Ignore it

☐ Have a discussion about needed change in behavior
(discuss a future, necessary, logical consequence given the severity of the behavior)

☐ Implement a logical consequence (reminding your child of the importance of health before anything)

☐ Appeal to your child's inner wisdom (have a discussion with your child about what you have observed, why you are concerned, the change in behavior expected)

☐ Reverse Time-Out (you leave)

☐ Group Time-Out (everyone leaves for 10 minutes)

☐ Regrouping (family meeting to get out of power struggle)

☐ Humor

My Plan:

Would a discussion be a good idea?

Heathy Coping Strategy I will address with my child this week and my plan to address it.

Express negative emotions effectively	Ask for more help	Set more limits (cut down study time, set a regular bedtime, cut out an activity)
Express an opinion- even if someone may disagree	Be more considerate of others	Place more realistic demands on oneself (consider the cost, not whether the demands are achieved)
Get a better balance of work and leisure	View a situation with curiosity rather than with criticism	Manage disappointing results
Share a vulnerability with someone	Embrace and learn from mistakes rather than running from them	Resolve a conflict
Tune in and respond more to what your feelings are telling you	Take more pride in oneself (being a more respectful self-parent)	Strut
Be Silly or just take yourself less seriously	Smile at your reflection	Initiate plans
Try something new	Get Messy	Break a ritual
Get more sleep	Other	Other

Possible Suggestions:	**My Plan:**
☐ Positive attention when takes a step toward behavior ☐ One-on-one time outside of eating disorder stuff ☐ Earning a logical privilege given increased health ☐ Praise and STOP – no BUTS ☐ Role Model Behavior Yourself ☐ Open the door for a discussion ☐ Set a limit ☐ Offer to teach ☐ Other	

Heathy Coping Strategy I will Role Model this week.

Possible Suggestions:	**My Plan:**
☐ Delegate something. ☐ Say 'no' to some things. ☐ Be honest with my feelings. ☐ Express my feelings when not on the wave. ☐ Ask for help. ☐ Set healthy limits between my needs and those of others. ☐ Listen with full attention. ☐ Praise and STOP. ☐ Say "I'm sorry" with no excuses. ☐ Allow family members to make mistakes without jumping in. ☐ Be consistent. ☐ Address negative self-talk. ☐ Be reliable.	

Self-care Strategy I will implement this week

Possible Suggestions:	**My Plan:**
☐ Make regular mealtimes a priority. ☐ Set a regular bedtime. ☐ Learn a new hobby. ☐ Spend some time with my friends. ☐ Spend time ALONE with my spouse. ☐ Set a regular time I stop work each day. ☐ Take weekends off. ☐ Buy something for myself. ☐ Exercise in a MODERATE manner. ☐ Take pride in my physical appearance.	No lame excuses!!

TIP OF THE WEEK: Always learn.

CHAPTER FIFTEEN: Communication

Where You Are

✓ You are an expert. We are fine tuning.

Congratulations!

Key Messages

It's a process: try, tweak, learn, grow.

"Self-parenting" is a necessary step for "other parenting."

Stay off the WAVE.

Remain genuine.

Topic: Listening

Communication is essential for healthy relationships. That's why you'll be happy to know that we have been working on communication all throughout this program. However, it is important that we make sure you have the key principles. They can be a bit tricky.

The most difficult part of communicating (in my opinion) is listening. Parents seem to agree with me. Listening is often the skill parents choose to work on for their homework. Many people **think** they are good listeners. However, even if you are pretty good, we all could use practice. Usually people who thought they were good listeners come to realize they have a lot to learn when it comes to listening. Ready? Here are the tricks.

1. Use your process approach and listen for understanding.

To really be a good listener, you have to be listening. Although this may seem obvious, it really isn't. Listening involves being in the moment. Your only goal for that moment is to **listen for understanding.** This is different than just listening. "Just listening" is hearing what the other person says. "Listening for understanding" is really trying to hear and **understand** the person's perspective. Many people get confused by the idea of understanding. Understanding is very different than agreeing. In fact, understanding needs a tip box.

Tip Box

No one shares the same perspective. The unique perspective of every individual is a result of each person's life experiences, beliefs and values, age, what captures her attention and on and on. As a result, the world each of us sees is different. None of us can **know** what another person is feeling or what they are experiencing. What we can do, however, is try to understand their perspective. We can listen to their view of things and try to understand why they have that view given the life that person has led. This does not mean we agree with her? It does not matter whether she is "right" or "wrong"; it is just her perspective. We have to be able to understand her perspective in order for her to be willing to listen to ours. It is very important for all of us to feel understood. Often we are not willing to alter our behavior or our beliefs if we don't think others understood where we were coming from in the first place.

When you are listening to another person's perspective, what you are NOT doing is:

- You are NOT thinking about what you will say next.
- You are NOT coming up with a rebuttal.
- You are NOT doing anything else.

You **ARE** listening and waiting for the person to finish. After the person has finished, then you can think about how to respond.

Tip Box

Good communication is like a tennis match that goes on forever with no winner. It has rhythm. It has turn taking. One person's move dictates the next move. Anything that disrupts this rhythm messes up the game.

---

2. Listen for feelings and ignore the fluff.

The goal of listening is to understand the other person's position. It is not to decide whether the person is right or wrong. Sometimes this is particularly challenging, especially when we think what the person is saying is totally untrue or complete nonsense. There are two different ways to handle these circumstances.

a) When we think what the person is saying is not true. Careful. This is trickier than it seems. We only see the world from our own perspective. Thus, sometimes things that seem untrue from our perspective seem <u>very</u> true from the perspective of someone else. By hearing their side, we can better understand how they perceived the situation.

Then again, you could be wrong. I know this has never happened before, but there is always a first time☺. Really listening means listening with an **open mind**; you are willing to entertain the idea that you may not have all the information.

b) When we think what the person is saying is utter nonsense. Ah, this requires expert listening skills indeed. Imagine your child is talking in "eating disorder speaks." Her conversation goes something like this: "I am so fat. No one likes me. No one will ever like me unless I lose a billion pounds." You know all of this is not true. You also know that trying to use logic will fail since she is clearly on the top of the wave. Now is the time for your secret weapon: **the content vs. process shift.**

What you do in this strategy is you totally ignore the content of what the person is saying, and, instead, try to listen for how the person is feeling. The tricky part is she won't say how she is feeling; you have to reason it out based on what is being said. You then focus on her feelings and the conversation goes from there. Here is what it looks like. It's easier than it sounds.

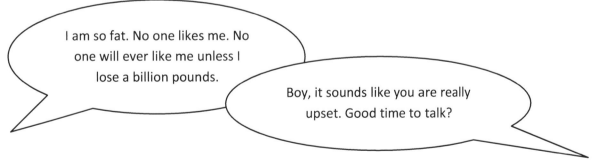

This clever parent avoided a daughter's outburst (her weight). In fact, arguing with her daughter about the content would have been very unhelpful and frustrating because her daughter was on the wave. Instead, the parent focused on how her child was feeling. This strategy has the added bonus of helping her daughter get better at recognizing the connection between her eating disorder symptoms and her true feelings.

Topic: Getting Credit for Listening

Imagine you have just spent all your patience being an attentive listener. There have been several occasions when you wanted to interrupt the other person with a "but, but, but", but you used all your energy to hold your tongue and really listen carefully until the other person finished. You even tried to listen for understanding. It is important that the other person knows you did this. You need to get credit for listening. This is crucial for good communication. If the other person THINKS you weren't listening (even if you were), then they will be less likely to listen to you and you both will start a vicious negative "non-listening" cycle.

How do you show the other person you've been listening? Well, you **act** like you are listening, you comment on what they said, and you show you are trying to understand their position. All these features are important.

1) Act like you're listening.

You may be an expert multi-tasker. You may be able to talk on the phone, balance your checkbook, and floss your teeth all at the same time. It doesn't matter. Even if you CAN do something else and still listen, it doesn't look that way to the other person. In order for the other person to think you're listening, you have to LOOK at them. You have to move your position so your body is facing them. If you are on the phone when talking to someone else, you need to STOP doing other things while you are talking on the phone. You may think you're fooling people, but you're not. People can hear it when you type while talking, or doing dishes, or drilling, or whatever. Just STOP. This communicates to the other person that you are giving him all your attention. This is incredibly respectful.

2) Show what you have learned.

Even if you are **acting** like you're listening, the only way someone **knows** you are listening is if you follow-up what they say with something **about** what they just said. This may seem obvious, but many of us just "continue where we left off" without acknowledging what the other person just said. You very well may have heard every single word, but they would have **no idea** of this.

Here's what **not** to do.

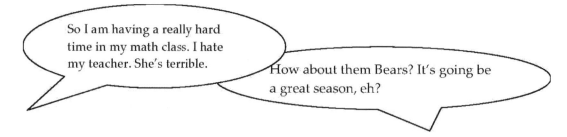

You get the point. Even if this parent heard every word, his child has no idea.

3) Show that you are trying to understand their position.

Your job doesn't stop there. While commenting on what you just heard shows you heard them, it doesn't communicate **listening for understanding.** You do that by trying one of these strategies:

Tip Box

• Ask a question to clarify what you think you heard.

• Summarize the person's position and ask if you got it right.

• Ask a question that gets more information related to what the person said.

Why do these strategies communicate you are trying to understand their position? Well, they show you are interested in what the person is saying and that you are trying to learn more.

Here is what **NOT** to do.

> So I am having a really hard time in my math class. I hate my teacher. She's terrible.

> What are you talking about? You are getting an A+ in that class. She can't be that bad.

Well, this parent is missing the point entirely. Whatever the **facts** (i.e. the child is getting a really good grade), the child **feels** like he is struggling. Thus, this is a perfect time to listen for understanding. It may look like this:

> So I am having a really hard time in my math class. I hate my teacher. She's terrible.

> I'm confused. You're doing well in that class. Do you feel like you have to work harder than you usually do?

OR

> What is it about your teacher that makes her so bad?

OR

> Are you venting or can I help? I used to be pretty good in math, you know.

Topic: Starting a Conversation

How about when **we** have something to say? When we need to talk to someone, we usually have an opinion regarding what we would like to happen when the interaction is over (although we don't usually give this a lot of thought). For example, we may want the other person to like us or feel good about our relationship when the conversation is over. We may want the other person to understand our position. We may call a friend for support and want to feel O.K. that we called her to talk when the conversation is over. Maybe we need a favor from someone. Thus, when we are done interacting with them, we hope that they will grant the favor.

Despite this goal, for our conversation to be effective, we need to stay in the moment. In any conversation, we only control our own behavior. We can't control what other people do or how other people feel. Thus, even though we may be the most effective communicator ever, the other person may still act like a jerk. **However,** there are things that we can do and ways that we can act that can INCREASE the likelihood that the interaction will turn out the way we want it to. Here are five quick tips.

Rule #1: Timing is everything.

There are good times to talk and not so good times. When people are on top of the wave, it is NOT a good time to talk. It won't go well. I promise. Instead, it's probably better to state your desire to discuss the issue later when you are both calm.

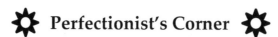

❀ Perfectionist's Corner ❀

<u>Perfectionist:</u>   But my child **<u>never</u>** wants to talk. What do I do then?
<u>Voice of Reason:</u>   Good point. Because your children may not be good at managing their emotions, they may try to avoid talking about upsetting things. It's still not a great idea to try to have a conversation at the top of the wave. A good strategy is to emphasize the importance of talking about it and reassuring your child that the door is open when they are ready to talk. **However,** if there is something that is essential to discuss, make it a multiple choice option. "Look we really need to discuss xxxxxx. We can either do it

tonight, now, or tomorrow morning. You choose." The message is that the topic needs to be but your child can have a say as to when.

Rule #2: Take the direct route.

The more direct and specific you are with others, the more likely it is that people may grant your wishes. It is hard to grant someone's wish if you are confused about what they want, right?

Rule #3. Agree with what is true, but don't sacrifice self-respect.

When people are on top of the wave, they can say a lot of things they don't mean. Usually these things are based on a small kernel of truth, but that kernel gets highly exaggerated when we are emotional. Your job is to ignore the exaggeration (this is very hard) and try to find the one valid piece of feedback the person gave. Take responsibility for mistakes you have made, apologize and move on. However, don't take responsibility for what you haven't done. In turn, tell people about things they have done that have hurt your feelings. Forgive and move on. The point? Don't get stuck. Stay in motion by learning and growing from each interaction.

Tip Box

So what are some barriers to good communication? Well, our **nonverbal** behavior; Things like our body language, our tone of voice, our facial expressions, our gestures. It doesn't matter what we **say** if our nonverbal behavior **doesn't match.** When our words and our behavior don't match, actions have a lot more impact. To make sure you don't suffer from **"nonverbal interference,"** become more aware of your nonverbals.

We learn how to speak, act, and communicate from those around us. We may have picked up some unhelpful habits along the way. What makes this more challenging is that we can't watch ourselves. Thus, it is VERY HARD to know how we come across. For example, a friend gave me feedback a while ago that I usually have a scowl on my face (apparently I scowl when I am thinking about things). Well, I had no idea! This feedback gave me the opportunity to work on this as having a scowl on one's face is not very welcoming (particularly when one is a psychologist)!

So, how can you become more aware of the signals you give off? Well, you are good at getting feedback now, so maybe ask a trusted friend or family member. I have even had some parents tape record themselves so they could listen how they come across. Then, you know what comes next. If you get feedback that something needs working on, make a plan to address it.

> Hey, I am trying to work on my communication. Can you give me some feedback on how I come across?

> Yeah, I'm glad you asked. Did you know you usually walk around with your eyes closed? Just thought it might be nice for you to see things once in a while.

Key Points.

1. Listening is a lot harder than you think. Make sure it is all that you are doing.
2. Get credit for listening. The other person doesn't know you've been listening unless you prove it.
3. Listen for understanding and listen for feelings.

Questions and Answers.

Q: Why is communicating so hard?

A: It can be hard, can't it? If it makes you feel better, it usually feels really difficult in the beginning because you are trying to learn new habits and to unlearn old habits. This takes a lot of attention and energy. However, once the new behaviors become a habit, it gets a lot easier. Genuine communication actually makes things a lot easier because there is no game playing. You know where people stand.

My Gift to Myself

Appreciate moments. Stop and enjoy moments of silence.

GOALS FOR WEEK #15

Date:

Remember our key guidelines
It's a process! Try, tweak, grow and learn.
Self-parenting: a necessary prerequisite for other parenting.
Learn how to SURF The WAVE!
Remain genuine.

Unhealthy or unhelpful behavior I will discuss WITH my child this week and our plan to address it.

Eats too little	Eats too little variety	Exercises too much
Throws up after meals	Doesn't get enough sleep	Doesn't set limits
Abuses laxatives	Engages in self-harm	Other

Possible Suggestions of How to Address:

☐ Ignore it

☐ Have a discussion about needed change in behavior
   (discuss a future, necessary, logical consequence given the severity of the behavior)

☐ Implement a logical consequence (reminding your child of the importance of health before anything)

☐ Appeal to your child's inner wisdom (have a discussion with your child about what you have observed, why you are concerned, the change in behavior expected)

☐ Reverse Time-Out (you leave)

☐ Group Time-Out (everyone leaves for 10 minutes)

☐ Regrouping (family meeting to get out of power struggle)

☐ Humor

My Plan:

Would a discussion be a good idea?

Heathy Coping Strategy I will address with my child this week and my plan to address it.

Express negative emotions effectively	Ask for more help	Set more limits (cut down study time, set a regular bedtime, cut out an activity)
Express an opinion- even if someone may disagree	Be more considerate of others	Place more realistic demands on oneself (consider the cost, not whether the demands are achieved)
Get a better balance of work and leisure	View a situation with curiosity rather than with criticism	Manage disappointing results
Share a vulnerability with someone	Embrace and learn from mistakes rather than running from them	Resolve a conflict
Tune in and respond more to what your feelings are telling you	Take more pride in oneself (being a more respectful self-parent)	Strut
Be Silly or just take yourself less seriously	Smile at your reflection	Initiate plans
Try something new	Get Messy	Break a ritual
Get more sleep	Other	Other

Possible Suggestions:	**My Plan:**
☐ Positive attention when takes a step toward behavior	
☐ One-on-one time outside of eating disorder stuff	
☐ Earning a logical privilege given increased health	
☐ Praise and STOP – no BUTS	
☐ Role Model Behavior Yourself	
☐ Open the door for a discussion	
☐ Set a limit	
☐ Offer to teach	
☐ Other	

Heathy Coping Strategy I will Role Model this week.

Possible Suggestions:	**My Plan:**
☐ Delegate something.	
☐ Say 'no' to some things.	
☐ Be honest with my feelings.	
☐ Express my feelings when not on the wave.	
☐ Ask for help.	
☐ Set healthy limits between my needs and those of others.	
☐ Listen with full attention.	
☐ Praise and STOP.	
☐ Say "I'm sorry" with no excuses.	
☐ Allow family members to make mistakes without jumping in.	
☐ Be consistent.	
☐ Address negative self-talk.	
☐ Be reliable.	

Self-care Strategy I will implement this week

Possible Suggestions:	**My Plan:**
☐ Make regular mealtimes a priority.	
☐ Set a regular bedtime.	
☐ Learn a new hobby.	
☐ Spend some time with my friends.	
☐ Spend time ALONE with my spouse.	
☐ Set a regular time I stop work each day.	
☐ Take weekends off.	
☐ Buy something for myself.	
☐ Exercise in a MODERATE manner.	
☐ Take pride in my physical appearance.	No lame excuses!!

TIP OF THE WEEK: Listen to what your emotions are telling you.

CHAPTER SIXTEEN: The Journey of Recovery

Where You Are

✓ You are at the end of the beginning.

Key Messages

It's a process: try, tweak, learn, grow.

"Self-parenting" is a necessary step for "other parenting."

Stay off the WAVE.

Remain genuine.

Topic: Recovery, what does it look like?

Well, now is as good a time as any to ask this question (although I am sure you have asked it many times already). It's a great question and I'll do what I can to take a stab at answering it.

The Journey of Hardship

Throughout this program, I have emphasized life as a journey with new experiences, growth, and learning occurring at each step. Evolution is a process. Illness and recovery are also processes. Just as your child didn't wake up one day and have an eating disorder, she won't wake up one day and have it disappear. Rather, the process of recovery is yet another stretch of this journey, a journey that has some notable twists and turns. I will explain each of these processes in turn.

The Journey of an Eating Disorder. I have talked much about your child having a "critical and cruel" coach inside her head (you may even have named this part of her). Well, if you stop and think about it, this has always been a part of your child (you may not have realized it because this is an internal struggle). Indeed, if your child often pushed herself beyond healthy limits, this part of her has likely been around a while. Well, the dilemma for your child is that, as a child, she was highly rewarded and praised for this aspect of herself. Teachers loved it, coaches loved it. You may have actually liked it too, because you didn't realize that it could be destructive. It's always nice having a successful child! It's always nice to have a child that not only listens to directions, but does more than is asked. To add to the confusion, she truly did seem to be fine. She was accomplishing things, and if you asked her, she said she was fine. You know now, in retrospect, that things weren't fine. Your child just had a limited ability to sense that things were not fine. Thus, the critical coach has been around for a long while, far before the eating disorder reared its ugly head.

This entire program has been focused on helping your child develop that part of her into a healthy guide. In fact, you have been working on the same thing in yourself. As you and your child have worked through this program, you have learned more about yourself, and your trust in yourself (and therefore likely your confidence) may be slowly increasing. This is not a project with a "due date" because this is not a process with an end. We can always be learning more about ourselves. This knowledge facilitates our perpetual growth. It would be both sad and boring to think that there is an end to this journey.

In fact, knowing oneself, trusting oneself, and possessing the willingness to grow as a person are but other names for the process of recovery. Recovery from an eating disorder requires two things to happen: 1) your child needs to learn to differentiate when her "self-parent" is giving her wise advice or unreasonable advice and 2) her self-parent needs to mature and evolve into the firm and supportive parent that you are.

Turning Point #1: When your child realizes/learns that she does <u>**not**</u> have to listen to that part of her, that any <u>**guilt**</u> she feels afterward when she doesn't listen will end more quickly with practice; and finally, that guilt in this circumstance is misguided. Your daughter is well on her way.

Turning Point #2: Your child learns to laugh at herself. She gets better at embracing every part of her; the quirks, the annoying habits, the weaknesses and the talents. She learns to value her uniqueness as a person rather than judge her worth based on what she does or looks like.

Turning Point #3: Your child gets connected. She gets better at listening to her body's messages and responding to those messages in a flexible manner. Such messages include signals of hunger and fullness, fatigue, need for relaxation, emotions. In fact, you have gotten pretty good at this yourself.

Thus, the essence of recovery is self-connection, flexibility, and acceptance. The goals for you during the course of this program are self-growth, self-connection, flexibility, and acceptance. Hmmmm... Your goals and the goals of your child are the same. The more you and your child continue to work on enhancing these features, the more comfortable you will be with yourself, the more solid your child's recovery will be, and the deeper your relationship shall become.

Putting It All Together.

I was struggling with the most effective way to end this chapter. Then a beautiful thing occurred that I had not planned (this is a true story). On the day I finished writing this chapter (or thought I had), a patient of mine came in announcing she had a college entrance essay which she wanted to read to me.

This individual is solid in her recovery, and I am exceedingly proud of her. I can't describe recovery better than she did. This is what she said in her college essay:

Evaluate a significant experience, achievement, risk you have taken, or ethical dilemma you have faced and its impact on you.

It was an illness that came at me like a tidal wave: first silently gathering momentum, then sucking me into its inescapable current, and before I could catch my breath, I found myself at the crest of its relentless fury. Just like that, it nearly slammed the life out of me, both in my body and in my soul.

You see, I believed perfection was within reach. Like most people who envision perfection, the state of flawlessness, I considered it the ultimate accomplishment. But what I did not realize was that it comes at a very high price, and in fact, it is a mere illusion that can never be achieved. For two years of my high school life, I fought with this allusive irony. I demanded perfection in academics, athletics, peer relationships, appearance, orderliness, and in manner. Perfection took on an importance above all else. It consumed me. There was no room for a mistake or fault. This impossible attempt expressed itself in the form of an eating disorder.

I have always been determined, as a perfectionist, to control the wave, no matter its size or force. I thought I could somehow master it. This was an expectation I held not only for myself but mistakenly believed others held for me as well. And while appearing happy, poised, and in complete control above water, beneath the surface, I was paddling frantically as the undertow of this illness pulled me into deeper trouble. At the time, I was unable to grasp the seriousness of my predicament. I began to lose myself in a battle for perfection. Meanwhile, the world around me sped by. I never felt the joy of the journey, or the satisfaction of achieving, because I always looked towards the horizon for the next biggest wave. Never would I allow myself to simply drift and enjoy.

By March of my junior year, I was sent home from my boarding school on medical leave. I left behind my school, my activities, my friends, and my three years of high school which I had come to adore. I came home, enveloped by the love of my family and the care of my medical team. After months of intense therapy, hard work, and daily struggles, I found a kind of peace within myself that I had never known. I learned to face reality and to accept that perfection is unattainable. Rather than striving for perfection, I now strive to learn for myself.

Retrospectively, this experience has been both crippling and strengthening. I am wiser, more self-aware, and more self-assured having confronted this illness. I learned an invaluable lesson through adversity. And for me, the first step in overcoming the adversity was to face and admit it. I am now confident that with a peaceful mind, healthful choices, and a desire to learn—for pleasure, not for perfection—my life will fall into place. Perfection is costly, but peace of mind is priceless.

This is recovery.

Where to go from here.

Congratulate yourself. You have seized upon your child's illness as an opportunity to learn. You understand emotions. Perhaps you have lost some fear you may have had about feelings. Hopefully, your life now has more balance. You may have become more accepting of yourself. As a result, you and your family are stronger.

It is my hope that your willingness to learn has been so rewarding that your first time through this program is only the beginning. We could all benefit from weekly reflection and goal-setting. I haven't included a weekly homework sheet with this chapter, as I leave it up to you how best to proceed. It is up to you how you conduct the next stretch of your journey. Please don't lose your spirit of openness, your respect for yourself, and your honor of relationships.

For now, I wish you clarity, acceptance, and peace. Your journey has now officially begun.

NEXT PHASE OF THE JOURNEY

Tip for Life: Enjoy the ride.

Remember our key guidelines:

♦ It's a process! Try, tweak, grow and learn.

♦ Self-parenting: A necessary perquisite for other parenting.

♦ Stay off the Wave.

♦ Remain genuine.

1. Think about yourself at the start of this journey with your child. How have you grown as a person as a result of your experiences so far?

2. Think about your comfort with your own emotions and the emotions of others at the start of this journey compared to now. How has that changed?

3. What about yourself surprised you the most? What did you think you couldn't do that you ended up doing?

4. Think about your family as a whole. How has your family changed as a result of this journey?

5. What would you personally like to be doing differently 2 months from now? What are some baby steps to get there (make sure these baby steps are things you can actually SEE so you know you are making progress).

6. What is something new you would like to try over the next few months? C'mon. Get a little risky!

Made in the USA
Coppell, TX
20 September 2020

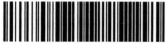

38418582R00157